THE LONGEVITY BIBLE

An Evidence-Based,
No-Bullshit Guide
to Living as Long
as Possible

JOHN ROSS, MD

To Leo McKay Jr., the better craftsman and the swellest guy

Paperback: 979-8-218-18837-5
eBook: 979-8-218-18838-2

Cover and book design by Mike Corrao, Mayfly Design

Library of Congress Catalog Number: 2023906691

Printed in the United States of America

Praise for Dr. Ross' previous book, *Shakespeare's Tremor and Orwell's Cough*

"A rollicking good story."

—*The Washington Post*

"Dr. Ross hits his narrative stride . . . in chapter after chapter. The stories of the wounded storytellers unfold smoothly on the page, as mesmerizing as any they themselves might have told, those squinting, wheezing, arthritic, infected, demented, defective yet superlative examples of the human condition."

—*The New York Times*

"[This] engrossing account of the illnesses endured by Shakespeare, Milton, Swift, the Brontës, Hawthorne, Melville, Yeats, Jack London, Joyce and Orwell . . . which deftly mixes close reading and diagnostic acumen, will stay with me for a long time . . . His light touch with cultural, social and political history is something from which many of the professionals in literary studies could learn. This is a book to which I shall return again and again."

—*The Wall Street Journal*

"Carefully looking at distinguished authors from a medical perspective, Ross blends biography, history, literature, science, and imagination in just the right doses."

—*Booklist (starred review)*

"Especially recommended for readers who enjoy historical context with their great books."

—*Kirkus Reviews*

"This lively, occasionally squirm-inducing book sketches the case histories of 10 writers whose health influenced their literary work . . . Into a satisfying series of medical mysteries [Ross] injects notes of wry humor and obvious affection."

—*The Boston Globe*

" . . . a fascinating, surprising, and at times hilarious compilation."

—*New Scientist*

"Most writers aren't doctors. And most doctors aren't writers. When the two talents coincide, readers are treated to rare wisdom and novel insights. John Ross skillfully walks us through a clinic of the famous unwell."

—*Nassir Ghaemi, author of* A First-Rate Madness *and Professor of Psychiatry, Tufts University School of Medicine*

"We always long to know writers better: more than just their words, we want to immerse ourselves in their lives, to really feel what they felt. This book does that, plunging you in the day-to-day pains and struggles of some of the most celebrated names in the canon."

—*Sam Kean, author of* The Disappearing Spoon *and* The Violinists' Thumb

"Dear sir," cried Sancho, blubbering, "Do not die—take my advice, and live many years upon the face of this earth; for, the greatest madness a man can be guilty of in this life, is to let himself die outright, without being slain by any person whatever, or destroyed by any other weapon than the hands of melancholy."

—Cervantes, *Don Quixote*

CONTENTS

PART ONE: UNDERSTANDING AGING

PART TWO: THINGS TO AVOID

PART THREE: THINGS TO DO

PART ONE

UNDERSTANDING AGING

CHAPTER 1

Time Out of Joint

Damage to DNA and telomeres is a major driver of aging.

A big clue to the mystery of aging came in January 1891, when a child in a mailcart was wheeled into the examining rooms of Dr. Hastings Gilford. The boy was only 14, but he seemed ancient and impossibly timeworn. He was wrinkled and bald, aside from a few white wisps where his eyebrows should have been. His head was freakishly big and covered in varicose veins. He had withered arms and legs and the flabby belly of a baby. With his wizened body, bulbous head, and bulging eyes, he looked like a geriatric alien.

Over the next three years, the boy became a familiar sight in Gilford's offices in Reading, England. Gilford could only watch as the youth suffered the progressive ravages of old age: creaky joints, plugged-up bowels, rattling lungs. Shuffling a few steps left him gasping for air. He had to sleep sitting up, because lying flat made him feel like he was suffocating. Oddly, as his body became decrepit, his mind remained clear. Gilford called his intelligence "uncommonly good."

When the boy died suddenly at 17, Gilford talked the family into letting him perform an autopsy. Gilford was shocked to find that the teen had the vascular system of a chain-smoking trucker. His coronary arteries were blocked, and his aorta carpeted with cholesterol plaques. His aortic valve was clogged with florid growths of calcified gunk that reminded Gilford of heads of cauliflower.

Gilford called the boy's condition *progeria*, which means premature aging in Greek. Progeria, thankfully, is a rare disease. There are perhaps 300 children and young adults with progeria in the world, or one out of about 20 million people. Patients with progeria all have a similar, slightly extraterrestrial appearance. It is one of those syndromes in which the patients all look very much like one another, while bearing little resemblance to their closest relatives. The prognosis in progeria is still grim. The average patient lives to be about 15 years old, before succumbing to a massive stroke or heart attack.

In 2003, American and French scientists found that progeria was caused by a mutation in the *LMNA* gene, which results in a defective version of a protein known as lamin A. In people without progeria, lamin A forms a scaffold that supports our chromosomes in the nucleus of the cell. (DNA, which contains the genetic blueprint for all the proteins in the body, is organized in long coils called chromosomes.)

By contrast, the mutant form of lamin A, known as progerin, gets stuck to the edge of the nucleus. A normal nucleus is smooth and round. In progeria, the nucleus is bizarre and misshapen, looking like a twisted potato. Without its lamin framework, the DNA inside is fragile and unstable. It soon becomes riddled with defects, which the cell is unable to repair. This problem worsens every time the cell divides. (The nerve cells of the brain stop dividing in childhood, which is probably why intelligence is preserved in patients with progeria.)

Cell division is a dangerous time for DNA, even in normal cells. Before dividing, a cell must copy its DNA, so that each daughter cell gets the same amount. Every cell division leads to a staggering 120,000 errors in DNA replication. Our DNA proofreading and repair mechanisms can usually correct these mistakes when we're younger, but our ability to patch up these gene defects declines with age. This random accumulation of genetic blunders is an important cause of aging.

The DNA in patients with progeria has another problem. DNA is like a rope made up of two strands. The ends of a rope tend to fray and unravel. Every time a cell divides, there is a tendency for its DNA to fray, with the loss of chunks of genetic material on the ends of its chromosomes. Nature's solution to this problem is to cap the ends with disposable bits called telomeres. Telomeres are like the little plastic tubes, or aglets, that protect the ends of your shoelaces. (If you are Canadian, think of telomeres as the tape on the blade of your old wooden hockey stick that kept it from splintering.) In progeria, the protective telomeres erode quickly, contributing to the ongoing DNA damage.

When cells sustain a critical amount of damage to DNA and telomeres, they stop dividing, and enter a twilight state called *cellular senescence*. Unfortunately, senescent cells are not meek retirees tending to their rose bushes. As we'll see later, they're more of a public menace, like your uncle with glaucoma who drives his Town Car home after an afternoon in a bar knocking back martinis.

There is another premature aging disease called Werner's syndrome. Patients are normal until puberty, when they fail to hit their growth spurt, and end up being the shortest kids in their high school graduating class. In their twenties, their hair turns gray and starts to fall out, and their skin thins and becomes easily injured. Patients in their thirties get cataracts, premature menopause, and osteoporosis, while cancers, heart attacks, strokes, and death are common in their forties. Werner's syndrome is caused by mutations in a protein called WRN, which—you guessed it—repairs damage to DNA and telomeres.

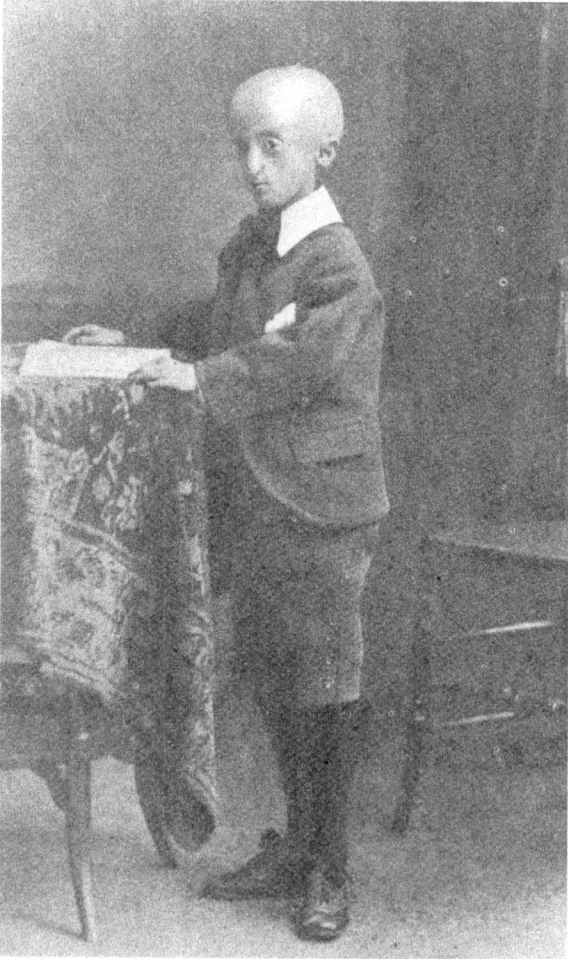

Gilford's patient with progeria, aged 15. Progeria patients suffer from premature aging because of extensive damage to DNA.

CHAPTER 2

This Cell Will Self-Destruct in Five Seconds

The body shuts down cells with too much DNA damage. This protects against cancer, but contributes to aging.

The patient—let's call her Gidget Jones—was having a rough go of things. She had been fighting lymphoma for over a year. Poor Gidget had been through an alphabet soup of chemotherapy—CHOP, MOPP, CCNU—but all of them spelled failure. Although some of her enlarged lymph nodes had shrunk after a new experimental drug, the ones on the left side of her neck had grown from orange-sized to grapefruit-sized in the past month.

Gidget is 13, but looks much older. Her back is crooked, her eyes are cloudy, and her ears are raggedy. The mitral valve in her heart is leaky, and she takes medicines for heart failure. Dr. Kristine Burgess shakes her head. "She's so old, she looks like she used to be good friends with Jesus." She greets Gidget affectionately and rubs the fur on her neck.

Gidget is a beagle. She is being treated at the Foster Hospital for Small Animals in North Grafton, Massachusetts, where Dr. Burgess is a veterinary oncologist and researcher. Gidget's parent (the word "owner" is avoided at the Foster Hospital) has brought her here from the farm in Vermont where he takes in rescue dogs. Dr. Burgess asks about Gidget's quality of life. According to Mr. Jones, Gidget is lively and active, despite her disease. "She eats well, she still tools around the yard. She'd be doing pretty well except for the baseball hanging off her face."

There is not much more to offer Gidget, aside from radiation to her massive lymph nodes. This would be a fairly complex proposition. Although the radiation treatment would be brief, Gidget must lie completely still, and so she would need anesthesia. Because of her leaky heart valve, the cardiologist has to clear her first, so Gidget is off for a chest x-ray and an echocardiogram.

Dr. Burgess's red hair is tied back in a bun, and there is a shower of freckles on her face. She tells me about the veterinary students from Tufts University who rotate through the cancer service at the Foster Hospital. "At first they think the whole thing is nuts, but then they think it's kind of cool." Cancer treatments in cats and dogs are better tolerated than in humans. "We give relatively lower doses of chemotherapy to animals. It's less likely to result in cure, but the side effects that people get, the vomiting, the hair loss, we don't see it."

People with cancer benefit from the study and treatment of cancer in animals. Many new cancer drugs are tried on cats and dogs first. Genes that cause cancer tend to be similar in humans and pets. These misbehaving genes are easier to find in purebreds, who have long stretches of DNA that are virtually the same from dog to dog. Amidst all this identical DNA, a mutant cancer gene sticks out like an albino at a tanning salon.

I admire a photo of a handsome golden retriever on a jet ski with its owner (sorry, *parent*). The golden retriever has had a front leg amputated for osteosarcoma, a common bone tumor in dogs. There are hundreds of these pet photos tacked up on the walls of the clinic. According to Dr. Burgess, many parents have stronger bonds to their companion animals than to other people. "All the time, I hear things like 'My dog got me through the loss of my parents,' 'My dog and I are getting through cancer together,' 'I lost my son, his dog is all I have left' . . . "

The cardiologist gives Gidget the go-ahead for anesthesia. The anesthesiologist asks, "This dog is not Addisonian, right? I just need to know that." Gidget is drowsy but still awake after a sedating cocktail of midazolam, etomidate, and propofol. "I'll top her off with a little more propofol," says the anesthesiologist. And Gidget is off to doggie dreamland.

Dr. Elizabeth McNiel, the radiation oncologist, gets ready. "Let's do a 10 by 12 field. Eight gray is my typical large fraction size." The radiation treatment only lasts fifteen minutes. Gidget is groggy and restless when she wakes up, but is otherwise just fine. Dr. McNiel is pleased, but not surprised. "Beagles are tough. They're a very resilient breed."

Cancer is common in the animal kingdom. Clams get leukemia, bulldogs get brain cancer, chickens get sarcomas, belugas get bowel cancer, and black-footed ferrets get breast cancer. Up to 90% of domesticated mice die of cancer. There is even a cancer of wild dogs, transmissible venereal tumor, which spreads through canine sex. A tactful scientist blames this on a "unique characteristic of sexual intercourse in this species that leads to injuries of the vaginal and penile mucosa and thus provides the bed for tumor transplantation."

Shark cartilage is a popular quack remedy for cancer, because of a false belief that sharks don't get cancer. As a result, shark populations have plummeted from overfishing. In fact, cancers have been found in 21 different species of sharks and in many different shark organs, including liver, kidney, lung, lymph nodes, and yes, cartilage.

Cancer is not just a problem in people, dogs, and sharks. Some bacteria and fungi hijack the growth machinery of plant cells, leading to the formation of bizarre tumors. Fruit trees get gnarly cancers called crown galls after infection with *Agrobacterium*. The charmingly named smut fungus transforms corn kernels into swollen, discolored blisters. Other plants develop cancers without predisposing infections. Karma alert: tobacco plants are especially prone to these spontaneous tumors.

You might think that cancer is a disease of the modern world, caused by our lazy lifestyles and nasty habit of dumping toxic crud into the environment. But cancer is actually an ancient problem, dating back at least as far as the Mesozoic era, some 200 million years ago. Duck-billed dinosaurs were strict vegans. They ate a healthy organic diet of puzzlegrass and rotten wood. They didn't smoke, avoided saturated fats, and got plenty of exercise running from velociraptors and tyrannosaurs. Yet, according to the fossil record, they were riddled with cancer. Scientists used a special x-ray technique called fluoroscopy to scan almost 3000 vertebral bones from duck-billed dinosaurs. Cancer was found in 1% of all the bones that they examined. (It is remarkable that we have any evidence of Jurassic cancer at all, given that we have only fossil remains, and most dinosaur cancers probably didn't involve bone. As well, most dinosaurs with cancer probably didn't survive long enough to develop advanced disease, as any major illness would have made them easy targets for predators.)

Cancer is not a problem for single-celled organisms, like bacteria and amoebas. But once cells banded together into porpoises, porcupines, and pangolins, cancer became a major issue. An amoeba can split apart into two separate amoebas whenever it likes. But cells in higher animals lose this freedom. They must behave themselves, play nice with others, and adopt a buttoned-down corporate mentality. The human body contains 37 trillion cells. Any one of them going rogue and turning cancerous threatens the existence of all the others.

Cancer is caused by damage to DNA. The DNA in our cells can be dinged up by chemicals, by radiation, and simply by the wear and tear of aging. Damage to two particular types of genes is associated with a high risk of cancer. *Oncogenes* make proteins that lead to cell growth and replication. These genes are very tightly controlled. In adults, they should either be turned off, or turned on only at low levels. If these genes mutate so the gene is always on, the cell is like a minivan with a stuck accelerator pedal barreling down the highway. It can't stop dividing and dividing, and forms a tumor.

The other kind of mutant gene that can cause cancer is a *tumor suppressor gene*. When these genes are working properly, they actually protect against cancer by repairing DNA or by shutting down injured cells with a lot of DNA damage. An example of a tumor suppressor gene is *BRCA1*. This gene codes for a protein that repairs DNA in breast and ovarian tissue. Women with mutations in *BRCA1* have a 60% lifetime risk of breast cancer and a 40% lifetime risk of ovarian cancer. The actress Angelina Jolie inherited a defective copy of *BRCA1* from her mother, who had died of ovarian cancer. Because of her high-risk genetics, Jolie chose to have her breasts and ovaries surgically removed for cancer prevention.

Evolution is so freaked out about cancer that it came up with its own version of Homeland Security, a tumor suppressor protein called p53. Think of p53 as being a cellular version of M in the James Bond films, a spymaster with a network of informers on the lookout for treacherous DNA. When p53 finds out about injured DNA, its first response is to dispatch a squad of fixers to see if the damage can be patched up and made right. If the DNA is beyond repair, the cell has two options. The first option is a forced retirement called cellular senescence, as we discussed in the last chapter. Senescent cells cannot divide, so at least they pose no cancer risk. However, they no longer do the job that they are supposed to do. As senescent cells accumulate, tissues and organs start to malfunction. Furthermore, senescent cells are bad seeds. They produce inflammation, and damage the healthy cells around them.

If p53 is truly alarmed by the state of the cell, it activates the nuclear option: cellular suicide. This last resort, in which the cell terminates itself with extreme prejudice, is called *apoptosis*. Once apoptosis is activated, the cell is on a one-way ticket to perdition. It digests itself, its organelles turn to mush, and it bursts into fragments. Both senescence and apoptosis are important mechanisms of normal aging, as well as premature aging syndromes such as progeria.

It seems harsh to have to accept senility and cellular *seppuku* as trade-offs for protection from cancer. But over the long run, there are excellent reasons for evolution to be really, really paranoid about cancer. One of these is cosmic rays. Cosmic rays are high energy particles that are born in violent galactic events, such as exploding supernovas and stars tumbling into black holes. Earth is continually bombarded with cosmic rays from outer space. Fortunately, most of these are deflected by Earth's magnetic field. Our annual radiation exposure from cosmic rays is relatively trivial, being equal to about four chest x-rays or one mammogram yearly. But there are times when our planet and our chromosomes are pummeled with massive amounts of cosmic rays.

On June 21, 2015, the Sun belched out a giant cloud of super-charged plasma, which crashed into Earth 40 hours later. Geomagnetic storms in the atmosphere jammed radio signals and led to spectacular displays of the aurora borealis in northern latitudes. Scientists later found that this electromagnetic spew, technically known as a coronal mass ejection, temporarily shrank the Earth's magnetic field, and even opened up a crack in it. This let in a flood of toxic cosmic rays, until Earth's magnetic field recovered two hours later.

This is not so unusual. These fearsome plasma bursts, known as coronal mass ejections, hit Earth about 30 times a year. Most are harmless, glancing blows. However, perhaps once every hundred years or so, the Earth takes a dead-on impact from a coronal mass ejection. The last time this happened was the Carrington event. On September 1, 1859, an amateur astronomer, Richard Carrington, recorded a mega-flare on the surface of the Sun. The next day, this flare landed a direct hit on Earth. Telegraph systems went down, as sparks flew from the lines and the contact points melted. The electrical energy generated the brightest aurora borealis seen in modern times. Colorado gold miners woke up, thinking it was daylight. New England farmers read newspapers by the light of the night sky. The northern lights were seen as far south as Cuba. A modern Carrington event could knock out satellites, fry delicate electronics, blow out transformers, and leave areas without power for months to years. As a side effect, it would also bathe us in dangerous cosmic rays.

Rarely, the Earth suffers ferocious and prolonged bombardments with cosmic rays. Earth's magnetic field is not fixed. The magnetic poles wander around, and the strength of the magnetic field has a disturbing tendency to wax and wane. Every half a million years or so, the magnetic field weakens and becomes more and more disorganized, and the North and South Magnetic Poles eventually switch places. While this is happening, the Earth loses almost all of its protection against cosmic rays. During the last Ice Age, about 41,000 years ago, there was a brief reversal of Earth's geomagnetic field, known as the Laschamp excursion. As a result, for 250 years, the Earth's magnetic field was only 5% of its current strength. Cosmic rays clobbered the Earth, leading to a high risk of cancer for any animals alive during this time period. It has been suggested that the Laschamp excursion might have finished off the Neanderthals.

Another reason for evolution to be paranoid about cancer is ultraviolet radiation. Today, the ozone layer in the atmosphere shields us from most of the mutation-causing ultraviolet radiation from the Sun. But before the ozone layer formed about 600 million years ago, life on Earth was mainly restricted to the oceans, where ultraviolet rays cannot penetrate. There was too much radiation in the shallow waters and on land for complex life to survive. The ozone layer made the evolution of large land animals like us possible.

At the end of the Permian era, 252 million years ago, volcanic eruptions in Siberia set fire to massive underground deposits of coal, oil, and gas. This dumped huge amounts of carbon dioxide and methane into the atmosphere, leading to runaway global warming. To make matters worse, the lava flows reacted with salt deposits, creating toxic chemicals that wrecked the ozone layer. As a result, animal life was bathed in cancer-causing radiation, possibly for as long as tens of thousands of years. Surviving this ultraviolet oven would have been impossible without extreme anti-cancer safeguards, such as senescence and apoptosis.

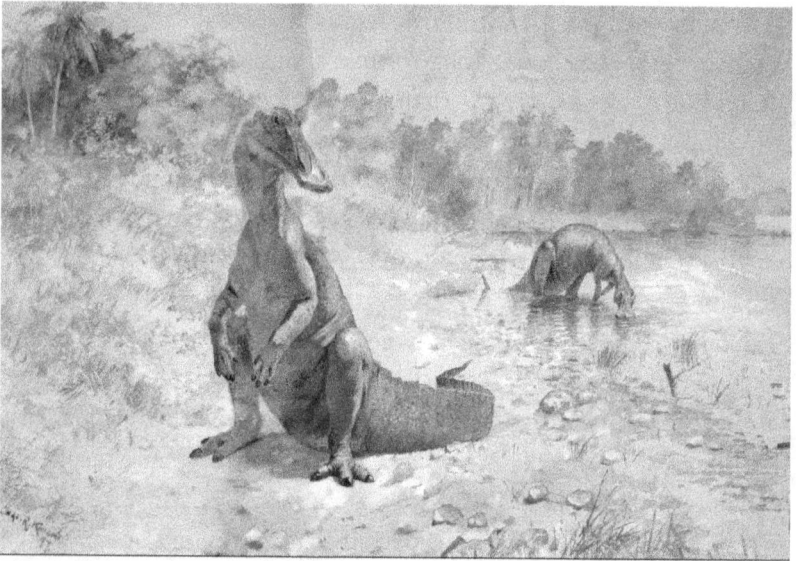

Candidates for cancer screening in the Cretaceous? We tend to think of cancer as a disease of the modern world. However, there is evidence of bone cancer in 1% of duck-billed dinosaur fossils. Evolution has come up with workarounds to reduce cancer risk, but some of these may have the adverse effect of speeding up aging.

CHAPTER 3

Clocks

Cells in the human body have a finite number of times they can divide, known as the Hayflick limit. In the short term, this protects against cancer, but in the long term may lead to a vicious cycle of accelerated aging.

In 1912, the French scientist Alexis Carrel discovered the secret of eternal life. Or so he thought.

Carrel was born in 1873 in the French city of Lyons. When he was five years old, his industrialist father died, and the family fell on hard times. This may explain how he became the type of abrasive, arrogant, and nakedly ambitious medical student that is now known as a gunner. In 1894, the President of France, Sadi Carnot, was visiting Lyons, when an Italian anarchist stabbed him in the abdomen. Carnot bled to death when his surgeons could not repair his torn portal vein. Carrel accused his professors of botching the operation, and set out to surpass them. As a surgical trainee, Carrel developed a method of sewing blood vessels together which later won him the Nobel Prize in Medicine. Much of his technique was filched from the seamstresses of Lyons, who taught him how to use the tiny needles that they used for lacemaking. (Carrel was neither the first man, nor the last, to steal the credit for a woman's ideas.)

Despite Carrel's undeniable achievements, he was blackballed from academia in France. This was partly because of his right-wing politics, and partly because he was a world-class pain in the ass. In

1906, he moved to New York, where he performed a series of organ transplants in laboratory animals. While this was pioneering work, it also displayed his strong flavor of Lovecraftian ghoulishness. In one experiment, he anesthetized a cat, removed its innards, and kept the disembodied heart, lungs, and bowels alive for hours by hooking them up to the vena cava of another luckless cat. Carrel also used his lab to indulge his flaky Darwinian fantasies. He built a giant complex of cages to create a master race of mighty mice. Some were fed well, some kept lean and hungry. Others were debauched on booze or exposed to poisons. Then the male mice battled to the death in a rodent Thunderdome: two mice enter, one mouse leaves. The survivors were rewarded with a harem of murine mates.

Carrel was a pioneer of tissue culture, the art of growing animal cells outside the body. In one experiment, he removed the heart from a chicken embryo, mashed it up, and placed the cells in a salt solution. Carrel claimed that the heart cells would beat indefinitely, as long as his assistants occasionally topped up the solution with vital juices from fresh chicken embryos. Carrel was skilled at milking his work for its publicity value, and his supposedly immortal cells soon became notorious. A sadly false urban legend spread that Carrel had created a throbbing chicken heart of monstrous proportions that threatened to burst forth from his laboratory.

In 1935, Carrel wrote a best-seller called *Man, the Unknown*. According to Carrel, democracy was a crock, the wrong people were having too many babies, and white folks were becoming weak and degenerate. Women were abandoning their sacred duty of motherhood to pursue kooky ideas about "education" and "careers." Society could only be saved by the mating of young people of high genetic merit. The feeble-minded, criminal, and insane should be euthanized. Countries should be run by cool-minded men of genius who abstained from sex, and were not tall. (Carrel was short, childless, and separated from his wife.) This racist and sexist farrago made Carrel an unlikely celebrity, and landed him on the cover of *Time* magazine.

Carrel returned to France just in time for the German occupation, and was put in charge of an institute devoted to carrying out his eugenic schemes. He and his staff examined French schoolchildren to assess their breeding potential, and bickered about whether North African, Armenian, and Polish immigrants were a threat to the French gene pool. When the Allies liberated Paris in 1944, Carrel was scorned as a Nazi collaborator, and died soon after in disgrace.

While Carrel's fascism ruined his reputation as a thinker, his scientific work was still respected after the war. His dogma that animal cells in tissue culture were immortal led to hope that human immortality might be tantalizingly close. Unfortunately, Carrel's science, like his politics, was heavily informed by wishful thinking, as the American cell biologist Leonard Hayflick soon discovered.

In 1958, Hayflick was a scientist at the Wistar Institute in Philadelphia. Hayflick had a theory that viruses were a major cause of human cancer. If so, perhaps he could isolate viruses from human cancer tissue, infect healthy cells with them, and make them cancerous as well.

Hayflick needed human cells that were unlikely to be already infected with viruses, so he started new cell lines using tissues from human fetuses. Hayflick's research got sidetracked when he noticed something weird. The cancer cells that Hayflick worked with were, in fact, immortal. Stick them in warm broth, and they would grow and divide forevermore. If Carrel had been right, the fetal cells should have also puttered along in perpetuity. But they were stubbornly mortal. The non-cancerous cells kept going until they had divided for about 50 times, then they petered out and died. Hayflick thought that maybe he was doing something wrong. He sent samples of the cells to other scientists to see if they could coax them to live longer, but the cells expired after 50 divisions for them as well.

Hayflick believed that Carrel had made an elementary blunder. Carrel had periodically added juices from chicken embryos to his cultures to encourage their growth. Hayflick thought these embryo extracts probably contained fresh cells that replenished the old dying ones. But the real reason for the prolonged survival of Carrel's cultures may have been even simpler: scientific fraud.

A scientist named Ralph Buchsbaum visited Carrel's lab in the 1930s in hopes of seeing the undying chicken cells. Buchsbaum also worked with chick embryos, but couldn't keep his own cell cultures going for longer than a year. He wanted to find out whether Carrel had a secret sauce that kept his chicken broth alive. The true man of genius was out of town, but a technician who was said to despise Carrel's fascist proclivities agreed to show Buchsbaum the infamous cultures. To Buchsbaum's surprise, they seemed to be moribund, with only a few feeble globules where he expected a luxuriant lawn of cells. Buchsbaum asked her how they could possibly keep it alive. She grinned maliciously and said, "Well, Dr. Carrel would be so upset if we lost the strain, we just add a few embryo cells now and then."

Hayflick studied other animal cells, and found that they too had an upper limit to the number of times they could divide. This ceiling on cell division is now known as the Hayflick limit. The Hayflick limit of an organism is a pretty good predictor of its life span. At birth, human cells have a Hayflick limit of 50 to 60 cell divisions. By middle age, our Hayflick limit dwindles to about 20. Mice, which typically live for three years or less, have a Hayflick limit of 10 to 15 divisions. The Galápagos tortoise, which lives as long as 175 years, has a Hayflick limit of 110 divisions. Cells from patients with premature aging syndromes, such as progeria, have a Hayflick limit as low as five or six.

Hayflick found that cells behaved as if they had an internal clock or timer that kept track of the cell divisions. He froze cell cultures of different ages and stored them in a freezer for several months. When he thawed them, they seemed to remember how many divisions they had undergone prior to the freezing. A human cell that had already divided 10 times before being frozen would divide another 40 times after it was thawed. A cell that had divided 20 times before freezing would divide another 30 times after thawing, and so on.

So what is this cellular doomsday clock? The answer will probably not be a surprise. It seems to be our telomeres, the protective caps on the ends of chromosomes that wear down when cells divide. After a critical amount of the telomere is gone, DNA damage and cancer-causing mutations become much more likely with additional cell divisions. When the cell's telomeres are too short for safety, the cell is forced into senescence, or early retirement, and cannot divide anymore. The Hayflick limit, and thus life span overall, seems to be related to telomere length. Cells with short telomeres have low Hayflick limits. People whose cells have short telomeres, such as patients with progeria and Werner syndrome, have shorter life spans. These conditions are associated with rapid telomere loss, as well as accelerated DNA damage.

An enzyme called telomerase can replenish telomeres. So, you may be thinking, the secret to immortality is adding telomerase to cells? Not so fast. In adults, telomerase is fully active in only two types of cells, both of which are theoretically immortal. Telomerase is found in germ cells, which perpetuate the species by giving rise to sperm in men and eggs in women. The other cells that possess telomerase are cancer cells, which need telomerase to reach advanced stages of growth. Dumping a bunch of telomerase into normal cells could increase cancer risk.

Evolution is all about tradeoffs. Because long-range survival is so uncertain, evolution tends to favor short-term benefits. The Hayflick limit is like an emergency hand brake that evolved as a protection against cancer. This is good in the short term, but bad in the long run, as it becomes a barrier to maximum life span. Furthermore, senescent cells do not go gentle into that good night. They're more like a gang of senile delinquents, smoking behind the old folks' home, shoplifting Geritol, and cutting water aerobics class to drag race their Chryslers in front of the YMCA.

Senescent cells simmer with malice, and poison their surroundings with proteins such as interleukin-6 (IL-6) that produce inflammation. High IL-6 levels increase the risk of type 2 diabetes, cardiovascular disease, stroke, cancer, frailty, dementia, and death. Chronic inflammation seems to accelerate aging, which has given rise to the term "inflammaging." Senescence can even behave like a zombie plague that spreads from cell to cell. Inflammation from senescent cells damages neighboring healthy cells, and may even provoke them to become senescent as well.

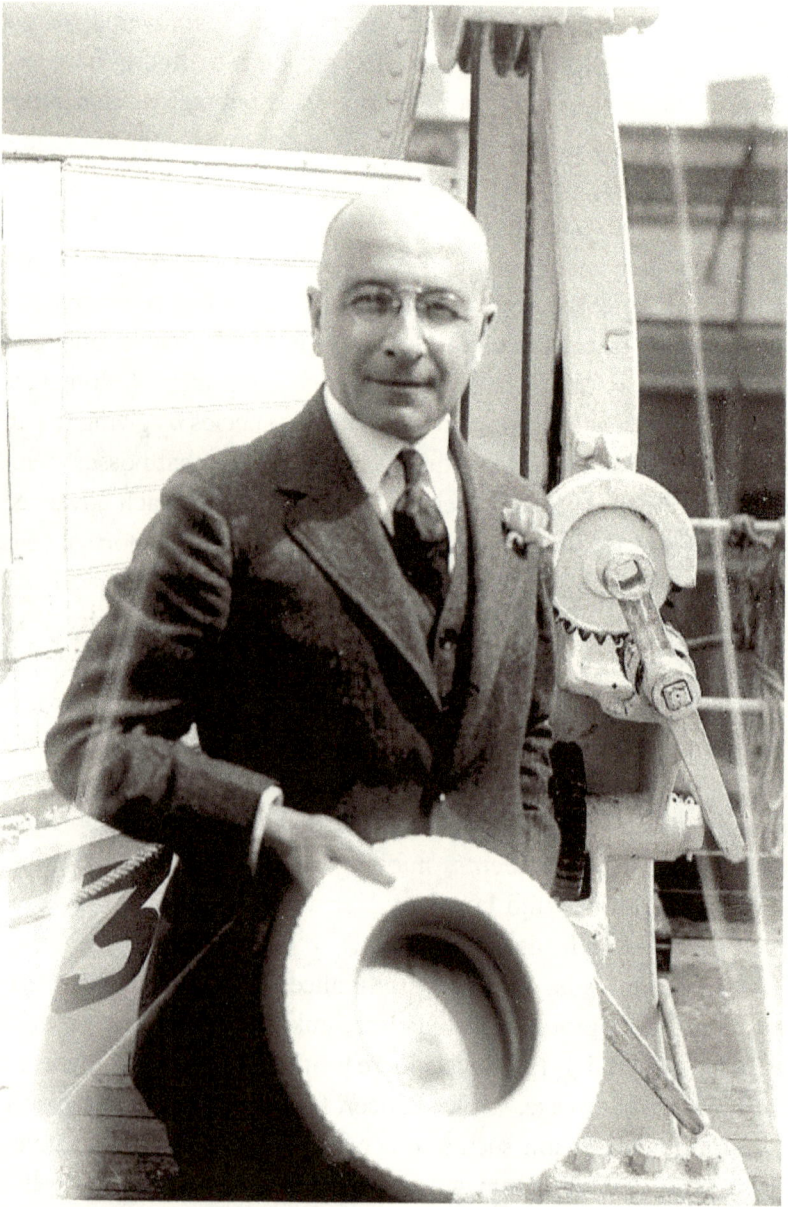

Alexis Carrel in happier days. His claim to have created immortal cells seems to have been an instance of scientific fraud. The life span of most cells is related to their Hayflick limit, which is a product of telomere length.

CHAPTER 4

Planned Obsolescence

Human lifespan, which is long relative to most animals, is limited by our ability to maintain the integrity of our DNA.

Our big job is to hasten obsolescence.

—Harley Earl, Head of Design, General Motors, 1955

In the 1970s, General Motors had a make of car for every make of American male. The Pontiac GTO was a high-octane steel cheetah for the young gentleman with more testosterone than brains. For the fecund family man, the Chevrolet Caprice Estate Wagon, a Mississippi River barge on wheels. For the doctor or accountant, a sensible beige Buick LeSabre. The Oldsmobile Delta 88 with its Rocket V8 engine was a social climber's car: civilized in externals, savage at heart. And at the top of the food chain, the Cadillac Eldorado, a chrome-plated Roman triumphal chariot, fit for a Dallas oilman or a Bronx mobster.

Aside from pitiful fuel efficiency, these gas-guzzling antiques had something else in common: they weren't made to last. The average car from this era only survived for five years on the road, compared to over 11 years for the autos of today.

Any scientific consideration of how to prolong life raises the question of why we must die at all. Why hasn't nature endowed us with a longer life span? Why are we doomed to the scrap heap, like rusted-out Pontiacs? Couldn't 3.8 billion years of evolution have produced immortal life? The good news is that evolution has already got this immortality thing figured out. The bad news is that it doesn't involve us not dying.

There is an unbroken chain of life on Earth, which probably began with primitive bacteria that emerged from the superheated waters around volcanic vents in the ocean floor. Our distant ancestors include go-getter fish that ventured onto land, sad-sack dinosaurs that turned nocturnal to avoid bullies and predators, and the first mammals, puny bug-eaters that lurked in trees.

All the animals that we descended from faced a daunting problem: how to pass along the best possible copy of its genetic material, or genome, with as few errors as possible. Although mutations are sometimes beneficial, they are more likely to be harmful. Human cells contain a total of six billion base pairs of DNA. DNA polymerase, the protein that copies DNA when cells divide, is good at its job, but not perfect, making a mistake as often as one in ten million base pairs. Our cells have mechanisms that can go back and fix most of these blunders. However, the proofreading necessary to produce an ultra-faithful DNA copy uses up a lot of chemical energy. As food supplies in nature are precarious, this expenditure of precious energy might hurt an animal's overall chance of survival.

Evolution solved this problem with an unsentimental compromise: to be exceedingly careful when duplicating germ cells, the cells that produce eggs and sperm, and much sloppier when replicating the cells of the body, or soma. In effect, evolution has made the cells of our germ line immortal, even if we are not. Tom Kirkwood, the leading scientist of aging who came up with this concept, calls this the "disposable soma" theory. From the callous perspective of evolution, the human body is like the stages of the Saturn V rocket that fall away into the sea when their fuel is spent. We are merely protective packaging for our precious germ cells, a carbon-based Brink's truck for the transmission of genes to the next generation.

Even though bodies may ultimately be dispensable, animals still need to survive long enough to reproduce and pass along their genes. There are two general life strategies to accomplish this. Animals may put almost all of their available energy into rapid growth and early reproduction. Newborn rabbits reach sexual maturity in three months, and mice reproduce in as little as 30 days after birth. Animals that take this approach typically have high mortality from predation. If you are likely to be eaten by an owl or a fox before your first birthday, it doesn't make much sense to invest a ton of energy into cellular housekeeping. So evolution has favored mice and rabbits who skimp on DNA repair and protein upkeep, and have lackadaisical immune systems. For this reason, their life spans are short, even when they are kept as pets and protected from prey.

The other evolutionary approach is just the opposite: a genetic makeup that delays growth and reproduction, and channels more resources into cellular maintenance for longer life. This strategy is both high risk and high reward. The risk is becoming someone's dinner, or dying from injury or disease, before you reproduce. The potential payoff, if you survive to sexual maturity, is that you may get many more opportunities for reproduction. Humans exemplify the latter strategy. Indeed, some men have used their reproductive opportunities very, very well. Based on studies of modern Y chromosomes, which are passed exclusively from father to son, three million men alive today are thought to be descended from the medieval Irish king, Niall of the Nine Hostages, while Genghis Khan seems to have left a staggering 16 million living male descendants.

While humans are long-lived by the standards of the animal kingdom, we are far from nature's longevity champions. Giant tortoises routinely live for more than 100 years, and bowhead whales for at least 200 years. The lifespan of the Greenland shark may exceed 400 years. This is good, as it doesn't hit puberty until it is 150 years old. Long life in these animals may literally be the result of good genes. Recent studies indicate that giant tortoises and bowhead whales have extra copies of genes for proteins that repair DNA, suppress tumors, detoxify free radicals, get rid of damaged proteins, make the immune system more vigilant, and mend telomeres, those fragile caps that keep our chromosomes from unraveling.

If the bowhead whale can live as long as 200 years, then why can't we? The answer probably lies in the evolutionary history of our species. For the vast majority of human history, most people died before the age of 40, with a few plucky survivors making it into their 60s and 70s. Under these circumstances, there was no advantage to the energy investment required for an extraordinary life span. Spending calories on DNA repair might have reduced one's ability to survive years of scarce game and failed harvests.

The longest-lived human ever was Jeanne Calment, a French-woman who died in 1997 at the age of 122 years. No man has lived longer than 116 years. It has been argued that, based on the constraints of our current genetic endowment, that maximum human lifespan is unlikely to be much in excess of these numbers.

The automotive industry has moved on from the short-lived clunkers of the Seventies. Cars today last longer because of tighter engineering tolerances, precise robotic welding, rust-resistant parts, fuel injection, and synthetic motor oils. Would it also be possible to genetically engineer humans with longer life spans? Yes, in theory. If our food supply continues to be as abundant as it is today, it would not hurt our short-term survival to divert more calories into preventive maintenance. We now have tools such as CRISPR that make it possible to tinker with the human genome, and plunk in more genes to boost our immune responses and DNA repair mechanisms, such as bowhead whales and giant tortoises have. For better or worse, it is probably inevitable that someone with oodles of money and a malleable moral compass will eventually try to do so. For now, we must make do with what we have.

CHAPTER 5

Size Matters

Being tall is associated with a higher risk of cancer death.
This risk tends to be balanced out by the higher socioeconomic
status of tall people.

You don't see many 7-footers walking around at the age of 75 . . .
most of us big guys don't seem to last too long.

—Larry Bird

Is bigger always better? Not necessarily.

In a seven-month period in 2015, six former NBA players aged 60 or under died suddenly. Anthony Mason, a starter on the Knicks team that made the Finals in 1994, had a massive coronary at 48. Christian Welp, a towering German who was a first-round pick of the Philadelphia 76ers in 1987, died of cardiac arrest at 51. Jack Haley, a surfer dude who won a ring with the 1996 Chicago Bulls, a team on which his primary role was Dennis Rodman's minder, also died from heart trouble at 51. Hall of Famer Moses Malone died in his sleep of coronary disease at 60, and former San Antonio Spur Jerome Kersey dropped dead at 52 from a massive blood clot. Beloved weirdo Darryl "Chocolate Thunder" Dawkins, known for his backboard-busting dunks and his claim to be an alien from the Planet Lovetron, returned to the realms of interplanetary funksmanship after suffering a heart attack at 58.

Intrigued by this spate of early deaths in ballers, researchers looked at life span and height in 3,901 former professional basketball players. They found that extreme height was associated with premature death. The tallest 5% of players in their study had the lowest average life span (56.6 years), while the shortest 5% lived longest on average (75.1 years).

Being tall was once a predictor of *longer* life span. During most of human history, when food supplies were doubtful and famine was common, steady grub, higher stature, and long life went together. Well-fed kids became tall, healthy grown-ups, while malnourished children became scrawny, sickly, short-lived adults.

But now, when more kids in developed countries are overfed than underfed, the relationship between height and health has become more complex. Several studies have shown that being tall poses significant risks for health problems and death. Taller people are more likely to get blood clots in the legs, herniated spinal discs leading to pinched nerves (sciatica), hip fractures from falls, and the irregular heartbeats of atrial fibrillation.

Perhaps most concerning is the link between being tall and getting cancer. Tallness in both men and women is associated with a greater risk of dying from cancer. Compared to short people, tall people have a 15% rise in the risk of cancer with every height increase of 10 cm (4 inches).

There are probably two reasons why height is tied to cancer risk. Tall people have high levels of insulin-like growth factor (IGF-1). This protein is part of a network of signals that helps to determine why people age at different rates. It stimulates the growth of normal cells, as well as tumor cells. IGF-1 also inhibits apoptosis, the pathway of cellular suicide by which the body rids itself of undesirable cells, such as cancer cells.

The other reason that tall people are more prone to cancer is simply that their bodies have bigger organs and trillions more cells than short people. More cells create more potential for things to go awry, and for cancer to develop.

This relationship between bulk and cancer is also seen in man's best friend. The largest doggos, such as Great Danes and Bernese Mountain Dogs, are also the shortest lived, with a life span of seven to ten years. On the other hand, the pint-sized Chihuahua may live as long as 20 years. At least some of this difference in longevity is related to IGF-1. Big dogs, like big people, have higher levels of IGF-1, which is associated with greater cancer risk and faster aging. (You may wonder how massive animals such as elephants and whales can be long-lived. The answer appears to be that they have extra copies of genes that prevent cancer by destroying tumor cells and fixing broken DNA.)

Although being tall seems to be consistently associated with higher cancer risk, not all studies show that tall stature is associated with a greater overall risk of death. One study from Hawaii of 8,003 Japanese-American men found that shorter height was associated with a small overall survival advantage. But in other studies, the lifespans of tall people and short people were about equal, because the higher risk of cancer in tall people was balanced by their *lower* risk of heart attacks and stroke, compared to shorter people. Although NBA-sized tall people are prone to some less common types of heart disease, such as hypertrophic cardiomyopathy, tall people have coronary arteries that are bigger, and hence less prone to clog up and cause heart attacks. Tall people are also less likely to have high blood pressure.

People that are tall also tend to get opportunities that the vertically-challenged do not. Tall people are more likely to go to university, and tend to have higher incomes than short people. Education and wealth are strongly associated with lower risks of heart attack, stroke, and all-cause mortality. And probably because they tend to have higher socioeconomic status, tall people have better health behaviors: they are more physically active, and less likely to smoke.

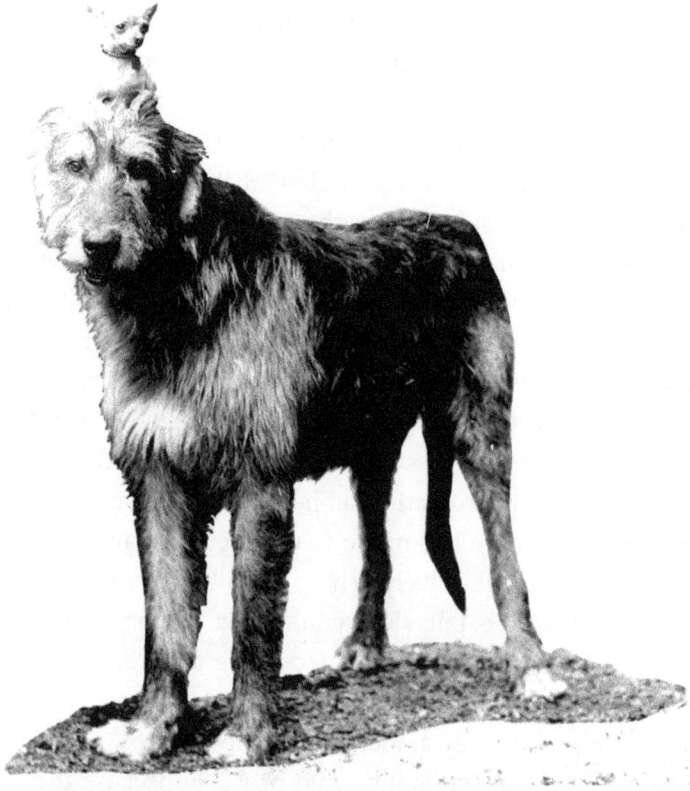

Dog show, 1920. Big dogs live for seven to ten years, while the pint-sized Chihuahua may live as long as 20 years. At least some of this longevity difference is related to IGF-1. Big dogs, like big people, have higher levels of IGF-1, which is associated with faster aging and a greater risk of cancer.

CHAPTER 6

Burning Man

That which nourishes us also destroys us. When we burn food through the chemical process of oxidation, free radicals are produced, which make our mitochondria age and break down.

Moneypenny: Have you got a mission, James?

Bond: Yes. I'm to eliminate all free radicals.

Moneypenny: Oh! Do be careful!

—*Never Say Never Again*

Once upon a time, living things on Earth got along in peace and harmony. Then a selfish and destructive creature arose, and threw things out of balance. The strange new species slowly poisoned the water and air with its waste. For a while, the environment was able to compensate and remove the toxins from the ecosystem, but eventually it was overwhelmed. The pollutants built up and led to a global holocaust, with catastrophic climate change and mass extinctions.

The time was 2.3 billion years ago. The lethal new organisms were cyanobacteria. And their toxic excreta? Oxygen molecules.

Before the evolution of animals and plants, the dominant life forms on Earth were methanogens. These were bacteria that produced copious quantities of methane, turning the air into a soupy pink fog. Methane is a greenhouse gas which traps heat in the atmosphere. This made Earth warm enough to support life, as the Sun was then only about 80% as bright as it is today.

The arrival of cyanobacteria threw everything out of whack, leading to what geologists call the Great Oxygenation Event or the Oxygen Catastrophe. Cyanobacteria used photosynthesis, harnessing sunlight to store energy in the form of sugars, and pumping out pure oxygen as exhaust fumes. The oxygen at first bound to iron in the soil, producing layers of red rock that persist to this day. When it ran out of iron to react with, the oxygen started to build up in the atmosphere. This killed off most of the methanogens, who like oxygen as much as vampires like garlic and holy water. Oxygen then reacted with the methane, breaking it down to carbon dioxide and water. Temperatures plunged without methane to hold in the feeble light of the young Sun. This led to the Huronian glaciation, the longest and coldest Ice Age to ever hit the planet. Earth came perilously close to turning into a lifeless snowball. And all because of too much oxygen.

Oxygen is essential to animal life. If you and I were forced to breathe pure nitrogen gas, we would pass out from lack of oxygen in 20 seconds, and be dead in about three minutes. But considered as an element, oxygen is grasping and malicious, the meddlesome drama queen of the periodic table, messing with its neighbors in a process called oxidation.

Atoms are surrounded by a swarm of particles called electrons. Each of the two oxygen atoms in an oxygen molecule lusts after more electrons. When an oxygen molecule reacts with another molecule and poaches its electrons, the other molecule is said to be oxidized.

Oxidation can be slow and steady (corrosion) or swift and explosive (combustion). Rusted-out cars in a junkyard are the result of corrosion of iron, and the Statue of Liberty is green from corrosion of its copper coat. Combustion, or burning, is the edgy, more glamorous cousin of corrosion. Unlike corrosion, combustion requires high temperatures to get started. Otherwise, you and I would be at risk of spontaneously combusting, and thus making fuels of ourselves. But even though we are not burning, it is true to say that we are smoldering.

Our cells use sugars and fat (and sometimes protein) for fuel. This energy generation happens in mitochondria, the power plants of the cell. Unfortunately, that which nourishes us may also destroy us. Oxidation in mitochondria mostly takes place in a controlled fashion, using proteins that contain iron to bind up oxygen and keep it from reacting with other structures in the cell. However, small amounts of toxic oxygen by-products get loose, like sparks from a fire. These are known as reactive oxygen species, or free radicals.

The body has defenses against free radicals, but they are not foolproof. Free radicals that are not cleared away damage normal structures in the body, leading to typical changes associated with aging. Free radicals also mangle DNA, increasing the risk of cancer. If enough DNA in the cell gets damaged, the cell responds by either committing cellular suicide (apoptosis), or switching into senescent mode. "Senescent" is a sciency way of saying senile. As we've seen, senescent cells are not harmless codgers, but bilious old men spewing inflammatory signals into the blood. This triggers a vicious circle of aging: inflammation from senescent cells leads to more oxidative stress and free radical production, producing more DNA damage, which leads to more dying and senescent cells, and so on.

DNA damage from free radicals is a special problem in mitochondria. These sausage-shaped engines of the cell resemble bacteria. In fact, they are apparently descendants of bacteria that were engulfed by our single-celled ancestors, and co-opted into becoming factories for them. Because they were once free-living organisms, mitochondria even have their own DNA. Having precious DNA so close to so many free radicals seems criminally careless and stupid, like storing the Mona Lisa in a boiler room, or bringing a Fabergé egg to a South Boston bar on St. Patrick's Day. When mitochondrial DNA and proteins get injured by free radicals, the mitochondria leak even more free radicals into the cell, perpetuating a vicious cycle of age-related decline.

Oxidative stress may be an unavoidable cost of living, but as we'll see, many healthy behaviors protect us from reactive oxygen species. Exercise may increase health and life span by building up our defenses against free radicals. A good night's sleep may help repair damaged DNA. The benefits of fruits and vegetables may relate to their moderate quantities of antioxidants. Conversely, although dietary supplements do about $30 billion in sales a year in the United States, there is no evidence that they prolong life. In fact, as we'll see, there is some evidence that guzzling industrial amounts of antioxidants may paradoxically be harmful. (By the way, some researchers believe that the role of free radicals in aging is overstated. They blame other sorts of cellular damage, such as protein misfolding, which we'll discuss in the next chapter.)

CHAPTER 7

Human Origami

Protein misfolding is a mechanism of aging that is especially harmful to the brain. It may drive the progression of Alzheimer's and other dementias.

"What is the secret of life?" I asked.

"I forget," said Sandra.

"Protein," the bartender declared. "They found out something about protein."

—Kurt Vonnegut, *Cat's Cradle*

In *Cat's Cradle*, a mad scientist named Felix Hoenikker inadvertently brings on the apocalypse by inventing *ice-nine*. This chemical is just water, but with the molecules stacked in a peculiar way, such that it freezes at room temperature. A seed crystal of *ice-nine*, exposed to regular water, prompts the other water molecules to freeze up, arranging themselves in the same formation as *ice-nine*. Hoenikker created *ice-nine* to make it easy for armies to cross swamps and muddy battlefields. However, because this is a Kurt Vonnegut novel, things go badly. A suicidal man puts *ice-nine* on his tongue, and becomes a human icicle. When his corpse tumbles into the ocean by accident, all of Earth's waters freeze, leading to the end of the world as we know it.

As it turns out, a major cause of human aging and death is cellular junk that is a fearsome real-life version of *ice-nine*. This lethal crud is called amyloid.

Proteins are long chains of amino acids attached end to end, like boxcars coupled onto a locomotive. They perform all sorts of different jobs. Some make up the structural framework of the cell. Some control the flow of ions and nutrients in and out of cells. Others send and receive signals to and from other cells. Some are enzymes, proteins that perform chemical reactions. But they all have one thing in common: to work well, these dangling strings of amino acids have to be folded up into the right shape. There is an astronomically large number of possible forms that a protein can adopt. Unfortunately, almost all of these shapes are wrong. To help proteins take on the proper structure, cells have over 300 "chaperone" proteins that stick to newly made proteins, and help them fold correctly.

Our bodies invest a huge amount of energy into proteostasis, or inspecting and policing proteins. Protein folding is a glitchy, error-prone process. Up to 30% of the proteins we make fold up incorrectly after they are made. These misshapen and misbegotten proteins are destroyed as soon as they are identified. Some proteins are notorious for their tendency to go awry. Mutations in the protein known as CFTR cause cystic fibrosis. The normal form of CFTR is highly convoluted, with serpentine coils and twists, and it fails to fold properly up to 75% of the time. Mutated forms of CFTR are even more likely to misfold. (Improving CFTR folding in cystic fibrosis is a hot area of drug research and development.)

Our cells have two major methods for getting rid of malformed proteins. In one pathway, damaged proteins are tagged with a small protein called ubiquitin. (As its name suggests, ubiquitin is found in all animal cells.) A banjaxed protein coated with ubiquitin is like a rampaging beast subdued with tranquilizer darts and marked for slaughter. These ubiquitin tags funnel the doomed protein into a proteasome, a barrel-shaped garbage disposal unit. The inside of the proteasome is lined with proteases, proteins that chop up other proteins. They degrade the deformed proteins into fragments for recycling.

The other major disposal system is the lysosome. If the proteasome is the cell's meat grinder, the lysosome is its stomach. It contains acid and digestive enzymes that break up defective proteins and other debris too big to fit in the proteasome.

Protein misfolding is more likely to happen when cells are exposed to free radicals, radiation, and heavy metals such as mercury, lead, and arsenic. Fever and heat stress also tend to jumble up proteins. (At a chemical level, cooking largely consists of breaking apart, or denaturing, proteins.) And as you might expect, getting older is another major risk factor for protein misfolding. Proteostasis, or the quality control system for proteins, runs down as we age.

Proteins that are folded into the wrong shapes may actually be toxic to cells. Misfolded proteins tend to form small clumps, known as oligomers. They also form long chains, known as amyloid fibrils, which look like ribbons with ripples on their surfaces. Both oligomers and amyloid fibrils may stick to the outer membranes of cells and poke holes in them. Cells with busted membranes spill out electrolytes, lose energy, and eventually die, if the leaks get bad enough.

To make matters worse, chaperone proteins bind to amyloid fibrils in a futile attempt to refold them properly, and wind up getting stuck to them, like a soldier entangled in barbed wire. As levels of chaperone proteins fall, more proteins fold incorrectly. Amyloid deposits expand and perforate more cell membranes, and a vicious cycle of injury ensues. With a critical shortage of chaperones, proteins that detoxify free radicals are likely to misfold as well. Free radical levels rise, leading to further protein misfolding. Cellular order is overthrown, catastrophic system error ensues, and the cell dies in a shitstorm of senescence.

Many diseases of aging are protein folding disorders. Alzheimer's disease is associated with abnormal clumps of two different proteins: amyloid-beta and tau. Parkinson's disease and Lewy body dementia are caused by misfolded forms of a protein known as alpha-synuclein. Amyotrophic lateral sclerosis (Lou Gehrig's disease) is associated with toxic aggregates of the TDP-43 protein. In type 2 diabetes, lumps of islet amyloid polypeptide accumulate and kill off the cells that make insulin.

In my work as a hospital medicine physician, I often see older patients who are still physically robust, but nonetheless suffer from end-stage dementia. Why do some protein-folding disorders affect the brain much more than the rest of the body?

There are two probable explanations for this. Mature nerve cells have a very limited ability to divide and reproduce. For the most part, you are stuck with the same neurons throughout your adult life. Other cells in the body can reduce their burden of amyloid by dividing. If a liver cell splits in two, each offspring will have only half the amyloid of the original cell. But neurons can't do this. The amount of amyloid in our nerve cells increases relentlessly throughout our adult lives.

The other reason is that misfolded proteins are similar to the seed crystals of *ice-nine*. Like leather-jacketed hoodlums corrupting a clean-cut teen, amyloid proteins can coerce a correctly-folded protein into misfolding and becoming incorporated into abnormal clumps and fibrils. Fragments of amyloid can even break off and spread throughout the nervous system. In patients with early Alzheimer's dementia or Parkinson's disease, this allows the disorder to infiltrate parts of the brain that were previously normal.

Protein folding disorders may impose a hard limit on the human lifespan. There is a protein called transthyretin, which transports thyroid hormone in the bloodstream. In the very old, transthyretin starts to form amyloid deposits on the inner lining of blood vessels, in the heart, and along nerves, often leading to heart failure, narrowing of the spinal canal, and carpal tunnel syndrome. Autopsies on supercentenarians, people who lived to be at least 110 years old, show that almost all of them suffer from this age-related (senile) systemic amyloidosis.

This all sounds pretty grim, but there are two strategies that may help fight protein misfolding. Our cells have elaborate mechanisms that measure the amount of nutrients circulating in our bodies. In times of plenty, our cells get slack, and don't invest much energy into upkeep. But when fuel levels get low, our cells wake up and realize they are under threat. They go into survival mode, fixing broken DNA and getting rid of damaged proteins, trying to stick it out until better times return. Not eating to excess sends your cells a message that they need to shape up and get serious about proteostasis.

The other strategy is exercise, which leads to low-level production of free radicals in the furnace of the cell, the mitochondrion. You'd think, after all the bad press that free radicals have gotten thus far in this book, that this would be a catastrophe. But paradoxically, the tiny spillover of free radicals produced by moderate exercise seems to be beneficial. The technical term for this is *hormesis*, the notion that things that are toxic in large amounts may be helpful in low doses. Or, as Nietzsche wrote, "That which does not kill us makes us stronger." (This did not apply to Nietzsche's syphilis, which did not make him stronger, and in fact killed him.) Like moderation in diet, exercise stimulates the cell to work harder at getting rid of amyloid and defective proteins. We'll return to these ideas in more depth later.

CHAPTER 8

The Weaker Sex

If you want to live longer, be a woman. If you can't be a woman, then try not to be a violent, reckless jerk.

Possibly no feature of human biology is more robust than women's survival advantage over men.

—Steven Austad

In 1846, the American Midwest was swept by a kind of madness. Mexico's grip on California was loosening, and yellow journalists proclaimed that it was America's sacred duty to seize this land of plenty for itself. Well-off, otherwise sane farmers rushed to sell all they possessed and join the wagon trains rolling west.

That spring, five hundred wagons left Independence, Missouri, headed for California. Several dozen wagons, with a mix of old Yankee families and Irish and German immigrants, fell behind and became separated from the main party. Needing a new leader, they chose a good-natured, but not overly intelligent fellow named George Donner.

Donner tried to make up for lost time by taking a shortcut through Utah that was recommended in a guidebook written by an adventurer named Lansford W. Hastings. However, there were major problems with this route, which Hastings had never traveled himself. The Hastings Cutoff, as the trail came to be known, was neither short nor easy. In fact, it was not even a trail.

The Donner Party slowed to a crawl in the punishing terrain of the Wasatch mountains, where a road had to be hacked through the woods, and boulders pushed out of the way. They emerged into the Great Salt Lake Desert, where they baked in the sun by day and froze at night. The wagons sank into the salt pans. The oxen, crazed with thirst, stampeded. Cattle and horses dropped dead or vanished under mysterious circumstances. By the time they reached the Sierra Nevada mountains in November, an early blizzard had brought ten feet of snow, and they found themselves snowbound. (The total snowfall that winter would exceed 22 feet.)

The luckless pioneers hunkered down in squalid cabins. When their food ran out, they chewed strips of boiled oxhide, and sipped broth made from horse bones. They were soon reduced to eating the bodies of their dead compatriots.

A group of fifteen, the "Forlorn Hope," staggered out on crude snowshoes to seek help. In addition to starvation, they were soon suffering from snow blindness and hypothermia. All would have perished except for the charity of some Miwok Indians, who shared with them what little food they had. After 33 days, one of the 15 made it to a ranch in the Sacramento Valley.

Rescuers were soon on the way, but they were hampered by monstrous snowdrifts and the poor state of many of the Donner Party. It was late April before the last of the survivors, a German named Lewis Keseberg, made it back to civilization. Keseberg had some explaining to do. He had somehow come into possession of George Donner's pistols and stash of gold coins. Moreover, he was found with a cooking pot containing the mortal remains of Tamsen Donner, who had seemed to be doing tolerably well when she was last seen alive.

After their horrific ordeal, only 48 of the original 90 members of the Donner Party were left alive. Women and girls were twice as likely to survive as men and boys. Those who were part of a family group were far more likely to make it than those traveling alone. In fact, 15 of the 18 single men in the Donner Party died. (As we'll see, single men fare badly in regard to life expectancy in general.) While the men of the Donner Party did more of the hard labor on the trail, it should be noted that of the fifteen persons who went for help as part of the Forlorn Hope, ten were men and five were women. All five women survived, but only two of the men.

Judged on life expectancy alone, there is no doubt that males are the weaker of the sexes. At every age and in nearly every situation, women are more resilient and more likely to survive than men. Women live longer in periods of abundance, and are more likely to get through desperate times of famine or epidemic disease. Compared to women, men die at higher rates in childhood, youth, adulthood, and old age. Male fetuses even make up a greater proportion of stillborn births.

As of 2016, the average woman outlives the average man in every country on the planet. In fact, male and female life expectancy is now close in only a handful of countries with a trifecta of dire poverty, high rates of maternal death in childbirth, and extreme gender inequality, such as Afghanistan and Mali. In developed nations, the female advantage in average life expectancy varies, but is typically three to six years. In Russia, women outlive men by a whopping 10 years, a difference that seems to be driven by masculine consumption of heroic quantities of vodka and cigarettes.

The longer female life span is partly due to hormone-driven differences in behavior and biology. Many premature deaths in men can be blamed on testosterone poisoning, that fatal combination of cocksure cluelessness and macho bravado that are the hallmarks of being young and manly.

Despite the 1960s sitcom stereotype of the ditzy female driver, American men are twice as likely as women to die in car crashes. Men are especially prone to get into motor vehicle accidents where speeding or alcohol is a factor. Men are four times more likely to get killed while bicycling, and ten times more likely to die riding motorcycles. Even on foot, men are a menace to themselves. Male pedestrians are twice as likely to get killed as female pedestrians, apparently because of their greater propensity to try to cross roads with high speed traffic.

Risk taking, impulsive behavior, and social isolation are more common in men. Men abuse substances, such as cigarettes, alcohol, and opiates, at higher rates than women do, and men more often die violently. In the United States, men are three times more likely to commit suicide, and seven times more likely to be murdered, compared to women.

A study of eunuchs who served the last Korean royal dynasty supports the notion of testosterone as an obstacle to longer life span. Eunuchs lived 17 years longer, on average, compared to other males at the imperial court. However, it is doubtful that castration would be acceptable to most men as a longevity strategy.

While testosterone may be a life expectancy liability, imbuing men with deadly overconfidence, women may be protected by the beneficial effects of estrogen. Estrogen lowers LDL, the so-called "bad" cholesterol, and increases HDL, the "good" cholesterol. It also enhances defenses against free radicals, ramps up the immune system, and relaxes blood vessels, reducing the development of high blood pressure. (Estrogen does have a downside: it promotes the formation of blood clots.)

Women have other advantages over men, ones that are hard-wired into our genetics. Women have two X chromosomes. Men have only one X chromosome, as well as one Y chromosome. The Y chromosome, which determines male gender, is a shrimpy remnant of the X chromosome, and contains far fewer genes. As a result, men are more likely to be harmed if their X chromosome contains faulty genes, as they do not have another X chromosome to compensate. This is known as the "unguarded X" theory.

Humans are sexually dimorphic. That is, men and women look different on the outside. Compared to women, men have distinct external protuberances, and are generally larger and more muscular. Males are probably bigger for evolutionary reasons. Being bulkier helps to defend territory, mates, and offspring. But size also comes with a cost. Men are programmed to channel energy into muscle and bone growth, and skimp on maintenance and upkeep, such as the immune system and defenses against free radicals. The male body is thus a superficially impressive, if fundamentally unsound edifice, like a suburban McMansion with defective fire alarms and a busted sprinkler system.

The news is not all bad for men. A man who lives to old age is more likely to be active and in good health than a woman of the same age. Paradoxically, although women live longer, they have higher rates of disability and chronic disease in old age. One possible explanation is that really unhealthy men just die off sooner. Another, not mutually exclusive, explanation is that being female has health downsides. Plummeting estrogen levels at menopause put women at high risk of osteoporosis. Women's wider hips and looser, more flexible tendons lead to knee strain, and predisposes them to arthritis. And while women are less likely to die of pneumonia because of their estrogen-boosted immune systems, they are more prone to develop autoimmune diseases, such as lupus, rheumatoid arthritis, multiple sclerosis, and Crohn's disease.

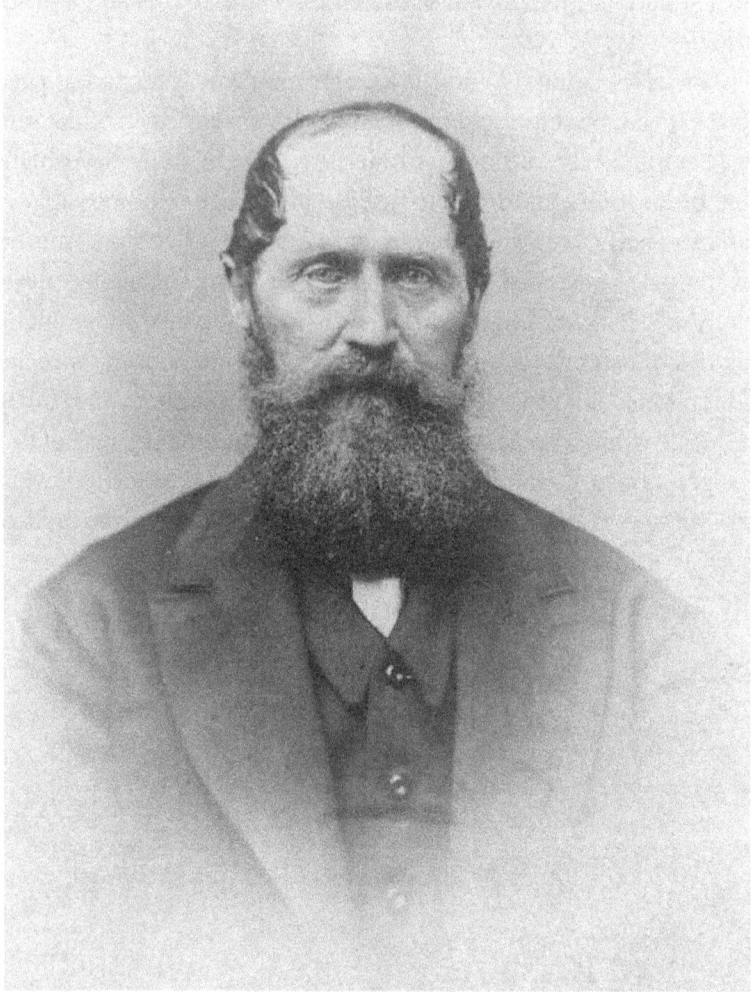

Lewis Keseberg, one of the few male survivors of the Donner Party. His survival seems to have been the result of skullduggery, rather than biological superiority. On average, women enjoy a life expectancy advantage of five years over men, likely due to better genetics and saner behavior.

CHAPTER 9

The Hunger Artist

Calorie restriction extends the life of lab animals by activating genes that shunt energy into DNA repair and cellular maintenance. However, this may not extend human life span, and could have serious side effects such as osteoporosis and frailty.

It's already possible to live to be well over 120 years if you start young and, as we shall see, take the necessary (albeit exceedingly stringent) measures.

—Roy Walford, *Maximum Life Span*

On September 26, 1991, four men and four women were sealed into an airtight complex of domes and greenhouses in the Arizona desert, where they spent the next two years dependent on recycled food, air, and water. This was Biosphere 2, a cross between a Martian space colony and a New Age sweat lodge.

Biosphere 2 contained over 3,800 species of plants and animals, and was spread out over 3.15 acres, about two and a half football fields. There were miniature replicas of rain forest, savannah, desert, scrub, marsh, and even a pint-sized ocean, complete with a diminutive coral reef. Half an acre was devoted to intensive agriculture, a trifling amount of land to serve as the primary food source for eight active adults.

Things went wrong almost immediately. The desert sky was unusually cloudy. The thick windows blocked too much sun, and they fogged up with moisture and scummed over with algae. Plant growth was stunted for lack of light. The bush babies devoured the hummingbirds, and swarms of tropical ants and cockroaches overwhelmed the butterflies and bees. Without hummingbirds, butterflies, and bees, the Biospherians were forced to pollinate their plants by hand. When mites destroyed the white potato crop, the crew gorged on beets and sweet potatoes, so much so that beta-carotene turned their skin orange.

Because of the imbalance between plant and animal life, carbon dioxide soared to unhealthy levels, going as high as 4500 parts per million, or over ten times its current level in the atmosphere. The excess carbon dioxide reacted with the concrete walls to form limestone. This took oxygen out of circulation, and prevented it from being recycled by the plants. Oxygen levels sank to those seen at the summits of the Alps. Extra oxygen had to be pumped in when the crew started to slur their words and develop rapid heart rates.

Their faltering food production limited the Biospherians to 1750 calories a day. For an active man, the recommended daily food intake is 3000 calories; for an active woman, 2400 calories. The average American takes in 3600 calories a day. The Biospherians lost alarming amounts of weight.

While most of the Biospherians saw the failure of their crops as a calamity, Roy Walford took it as a research opportunity. Walford was a physician who had written eight books and hundreds of peer-reviewed scientific papers. At 67, he was much older than the other Biospherians, and had led a colorful life, especially by the drab standards of academic medicine. In his youth, he and a buddy went to Reno, figured out which roulette wheels were slightly off kilter, and made a small fortune before the casinos tossed them. Their winnings paid for medical school, a house, and a sailboat in which they cruised the Caribbean for eighteen months. In the 1960s, he befriended LSD guru Timothy Leary, and dabbled in guerilla theater and performance art. In the 1970s, he pumped iron, shaved his head, hung out with punks, and gunned motorcycles down Santa Monica Boulevard. But his true passion was the prevention of aging, a pursuit he took to absurd lengths. Finding that fruit flies and lizards lived longer when exposed to cold, he became obsessed with human hibernation as a longevity strategy. He then wandered the Indian subcontinent sticking thermometers in the rectums of yogis, to see if the holy men could lower their body temperatures at will.

Walford had long advocated calorie restriction, or as he called it, "healthy starvation," as a means of life extension. The Biosphere diet was perfect from Walford's perspective: heavy on fruits and vegetables, low in dairy and meat, and dense in micronutrients (the Biospherians also took a daily multivitamin, just in case). It was low in fat, relatively heavy on carbohydrates, and had just enough protein.

On this spartan regime, the crew of Biosphere 2 had blood tests and vital signs that would be the envy of the average cornfed American. Their cholesterol and triglyceride levels plummeted, their glucose control was superb, and their blood pressures were impeccable. But they looked gaunt and emaciated, feuded with each other, felt exhausted and miserable, and their blood levels of pesticides and dioxins spiked up. These chemicals were banned from Biosphere 2. Where had they come from? The most likely explanation was that the buildup of these toxins in their body fat over several decades was washing out as they lost weight. There was another cause for concern: something had gone dreadfully wrong with Walford's walking. Walford, once a wrestler, gymnast, and champion jitterbug dancer, now tottered along with a clumsy, stumbling gait.

There is a long history of ascetic self-denial as a putative pathway to longevity. In ancient China, the student of Taoism who wished to become one of the *hsien*, or immortals, would hold his breath, grind his teeth, and eat only one meal a day, consisting of a few roots and berries. The would-be *hsien* would also manipulate his genitals during intercourse to provoke retrograde ejaculation, thus preserving his precious bodily essence. Rotten molars, hunger pangs, and a bladder full of semen were apparently a small price to pay for immortality.

Luigi Cornaro, an Italian nobleman of the High Renaissance, was so riddled with gout and peptic ulcers in his thirties that he was given mere months to live by his physicians. He stopped drinking, switched to a miserly diet of measly portions, got rich investing in Venetian swampland, wrote learned treatises in his eighties, and lived to the ripe old age of 98.

The modern science of starvation for health begins in 1934 with Clive McCay, a fast-talking Hoosier who was a professor of animal husbandry and nutrition at Cornell. In his lifetime, McCay was notorious for his startling testimony to Congress in 1950 that he was able to dissolve teeth by leaving them in Coca-Cola for 48 hours. But he is now mainly remembered for his pioneering studies of calorie restriction in rats.

McCay studied two groups of rats. One group ate as much as they wanted, while the other was fed low-calorie diets with adequate amounts of vitamins and minerals. The full-bodied rats lived an average of 509 days, while the underfed rats lived an average of 883 days. One famished rodent Methuselah lived an exceptional 1,456 days.

McCay's starveling rats rarely got cancer, which was common in the regularly fed rats, and they stayed active and kept their silky fur into old age. On the flip side, the scrawny rats had brittle bones and were undersexed and often sterile.

Calorie restriction failed to catch on, for one obvious reason: starving yourself voluntarily is no fun. As Leonard Hayflick observed, "In the 40 years since we have known about undernutrition, no one has consciously chosen to do it, even the biologists . . . any method is unacceptable if it affects the enjoyment of life."

Fifty years after McCay's studies, Roy Walford single-handedly revived popular interest in calorie restriction, with bestselling books such as *The 120-Year Diet*. Walford's own work had shown the best results with the most extreme diets. Mice fed only 35% of the normal amount of calories lived 67% longer than control mice. The starved mice had better immune function (at least in the test tube) and fewer cancers, compared to normally fed mice. However, the food-deprived mice were puny, and more prone to dying young.

Based on his data, Walford claimed that caloric restriction starting in childhood could prolong maximum human lifespan to 140 years, although he sadly admitted it might not be worth it, as the ill-fed kids would have stunted growth, and a few would die prematurely. While calorie restriction was most effective in mice who had just weaned from breastfeeding, Walford showed that it also prolonged life in mice when begun in middle age, although the results were less impressive.

Calorie restriction increased the lifespan of other species, including yeast, roundworms, and fruit flies. Intermittent fasting also seemed to work: rats that fasted every third day, but ate normally on the other days, had a 20% longer life span, compared to rats fed daily.

Although researchers knew for decades that calorie restriction increased life span, at least in the sheltered world of the laboratory, they had no idea how it worked. Progress was held back by the rudimentary tools then available to study the biology of aging, as well as the Dangerfieldesque lack of respect accorded to the whole field. For the scientific mainstream, the study of aging was a fringe endeavor, a disreputable realm of quacks and headline chasers, barely better than the quest for the philosopher's stone or the contrivance of perpetual motion machines.

The enigma of calorie restriction began to be unraveled in the early 1980s, when Michael Klass, then a cell biologist at the University of Houston, created long-lived mutants of *Caenorhabditis elegans*. This roundworm, more commonly known as *C. elegans*, is barely visible to the naked eye, but it has many advantages for laboratory research. It can be grown cheaply and in bulk on petri dishes at room temperature; it is not a fussy eater, and will happily chow down on an unappetizing diet of *E. coli* bacteria; it is transparent, and its organs can readily be seen under a microscope; it is hardy, and survives freezing and thawing; and it only lives for about 14 days, allowing for scientists to study the genetics of many generations in a short period of time. The vast majority of *C. elegans* are hermaphrodites, or self-fertilizing females, with males occurring in only one out of a thousand worms. *C. elegans* was the first animal to have its genome and its nervous system completely mapped out. True to form, 24% of the nervous system of the male worm is hardwired for sexual behavior, versus only 3% for the females.

Klass bombarded his roundworms with chemicals to damage their DNA, and screened the resulting 8000 mutants for long life span. Eight of the resulting strains were long-lived. Two of these strains lived longer because of arrested development: they failed to mature out of a larval stage. The other strains reached adulthood, and lived up to 110% longer than regular roundworms. However, they tended to be feeble and weedy-looking. Klass concluded, incorrectly, that their longevity was an indirect consequence of being unable to swallow properly, and that their long lives were really due to calorie restriction.

Klass thought that his great mutant hunt was a failure, and his papers were greeted with profound indifference by the scientific community. Feeling at an intellectual dead end, and distracted by an ongoing divorce, he left academia for the pharmaceutical industry, and bequeathed his wriggling greybeards to Tom Johnson, a former colleague at the University of Colorado Boulder.

Johnson, a Jesuit-educated redhead and Van Morrison lookalike, thawed out Klass' antique worms, and set to work. To his astonishment, Johnson found that most of the mutant roundworms actually ate just fine, and that their longer lives were really due to a gene mutation that slowed their rate of aging. Johnson named this mutated gene *age-1*. Johnson's discovery led to much skepticism from his peers, as well as an invitation to appear on television with Larry King, which he politely declined.

In the years since Johnson discovered *age-1*, we have learned that there are dozens of other gerontogenes, or genes that influence the rate of aging. These genes are deeply conserved, meaning that versions of them have been found in almost all animals that have been studied, including roundworms, fruit flies, mice, and humans. They seem to be part of a fiendishly complex cellular fuel gauge, an elaborate master switch for metabolism that helps animals to adjust to caloric boom and bust cycles.

In times of plenty, when animals are well fed, levels of insulin and growth hormone are high. (Growth hormone acts on cells indirectly, by boosting levels of insulin-like growth factor 1, or IGF-1). Cells get the green light to grow and divide, and energy is channeled into reproduction. But in times of scarcity, levels of insulin and IGF-1 plummet. Growth is halted. Starved cells shift into survival mode, like a doomsday prepper hunkered down in an Idaho bunker. Famished animals put the kibosh on sex, postpone reproduction until better times return, and invest in maintenance, fixing broken DNA, recycling defective proteins, and getting rid of free radicals.

Where does *age-1* fit into this? We now know that the *age-1* gene is the roundworm version of the human gene known as *PI3K*. This gene is the blueprint for a protein with the tongue-twisting name of phosphatidylinositol 3-kinase. PI3K (the protein, not the gene) is turned on when cells are stimulated by insulin or IGF-1. PI3K in turn stimulates another growth signal, AKT1 (a hyperactive *AKT1* gene is thought to have caused the deformities of Joseph Merrick, the Elephant Man). And AKT1 activates a protein called mTOR, or molecular target of rapamycin. (Rapamycin is a drug that suppresses the immune system, made by a bacterium discovered on Easter Island, the volcanic isle known to the locals as Rapa Nui.)

Greater activity along the PI3K-AKT1-mTOR axis leads to cell growth, a shorter life span, and a higher cancer risk. (In fact, many cancers arise from mutations that increase signaling in these proteins.) When it is less active, as in Klass and Johnson's roundworms with damaged *age-1* genes, or McCay and Walford's calorie-restricted mice, life span is prolonged. Strains of mice that have been genetically engineered with different defects in this pathway, such as decreased amounts of PI3K, AKT1, mTOR, insulin, or IGF-1, all live longer than normal mice.

If *PI3K*, *AKT*, and *MTOR* are bad actors from a life span standpoint, there are also genes that favor longevity. These genes, which include *SIRT1*, *FOXO3*, *PTEN*, and *AMPK*, should have the Good Housekeeping Seal of Approval. In the presence of cellular distress signals, such as low energy levels from calorie restriction, they help to keep the soma neat and tidy, mending worn-out DNA, scrubbing away unsightly free radicals, and hoovering up those pesky oxidized protein and fat molecules. (Scientists are trying to figure out if there is a way to turn these genes on without the nuisance of self-denial. We'll return to the status of this research later.)

The discovery of genes such as *PI3K* and *SIRT1* seems to have settled the mystery about the nature of aging. Is aging an inevitable accumulation of random damage over time? Is there some genetic control over aging? The answer seems to be yes on both counts. Aging results from gradual tissue damage from reactive oxygen species and other toxins. Different animal species have different life spans based on how much energy they invest in growth and reproduction, relative to how much energy they invest in repairing the soma. These investment strategies seem to be determined by genetics.

We know that calorie restriction in laboratory animals prolongs life. We also know that mutations in genes such as *age-1* extend lifespan by stimulating the cellular mechanisms seen in calorie restriction. So, shouldn't everyone try to practice calorie restriction?

Well, maybe not just yet. One downside is that animals that are calorie-restricted, or have genetic mutations that mimic calorie restriction, may be delicate hothouse flowers that only survive in the controlled conditions of the laboratory. Compared to their wild-type cousins, they are less robust and less fertile. In fact, Tom Johnson found that when *age-1* mutants were placed in direct competition with regular roundworms, the *age-1* mutants went extinct after only four generations.

Calorie-restricted animals also have more trouble fighting off infections. While their immune cells work well in the test tube, mice with longstanding calorie restriction are prone to develop overwhelming infections with parasitic worms. They are also more likely to die of influenza or sepsis than normally fed mice. This dovetails with the long and lamentable history of deadly epidemics during times of famine.

There are other potential harms from calorie restriction. Roundworms and fruit flies only live for days or weeks. Mice only live a year or two. A human being lasts for many decades, provided it gets proper nutrition, running maintenance, and a dash of good fortune. We already invest way more energy in basic upkeep than round-worms, fruit flies, and mice do. What works for them might not necessarily work for us.

For example, calorie restriction might worsen frailty, the loss of bone and muscle with age that leads to falls, fractures, loss of independence, and even death. For the elderly patients I treat in the hospital, a hip fracture is often catastrophic, leading to a downward spiral of complications such as pneumonia and delirium. About 30% of aging patients die within a year of having a hip fracture. We also have a critical organ that burns through a humongous amount of fuel: our nervous system. The brain consumes about 20% of our daily energy expenditure. Could our bones and brains become casualties of calorie restriction?

We have some evidence that sheds light on the risks and benefits of calorie restriction for long-lived primates like ourselves. There are two long-term studies of underfeeding in the rhesus macaque monkey. We share 93% of our DNA with the rhesus macaque, which lives as long as 40 years, so it is probably a better model of the effectiveness of calorie restriction in humans than Roy Walford's mice.

These two studies showed somewhat differing results. One study, performed at the University of Wisconsin, showed that the calorie-restricted monkeys were healthier and were less likely to die of diseases of aging, such as cardiovascular disease and cancer. However, they were perhaps a little more prone to die from other causes, and their overall risk of death was similar to the controls (the monkeys that ate as much as they wanted). By contrast, the study performed at the National Institute of Aging (NIA) was essentially negative, showing no benefit of calorie restriction in preventing age-related disease or improving survival.

What might explain the difference in outcomes between the two studies? The high rate of age-related disease in the Wisconsin controls might be explained by the unhealthy monkey chow used in that study, which was heavily processed and contained alarming amounts of sucrose. By contrast, the NIA monkeys ate a more natural diet, with soy, corn, and fish oils, and minimal amounts of simple sugars. If the NIA control monkeys were ponytailed boomers nibbling kale and granola from Whole Foods, the Wisconsin controls were simian Homer Simpsons, stuffing their faces with jelly donuts.

There is a study of mild calorie restriction in human adults, the CALERIE-2 trial. Weight, blood pressure, cholesterol, mood, sleep, and sex life improved in the calorie-restricted group. CALERIE-2 might be better described as a study of sustained dieting, rather than true caloric restriction. Food intake in restricted subjects was only 12% lower than controls, a piddly amount compared to the draconian 35-65% calorie restriction in Roy Walford's mouse studies. The major drawback was osteoporosis, with calorie-restricted subjects having small but significant declines in bone density. (Anecdotally, osteoporosis is a huge problem in serious practitioners of calorie restriction.) Finally, there is one other possible hazard of human calorie restriction.

After leaving Biosphere 2, Roy Walford continued to have trouble with balance and weakness. He struggled to stand, needed a walker to keep from falling, and began to slur his speech and have difficulty swallowing. He was eventually diagnosed with amyotrophic lateral sclerosis (ALS), also known as Lou Gehrig's disease, a disease of nerve cells in the brain and spinal cord that causes progressive immobility. Walford died at the age of 79 after a very full life, albeit well short of his 120-year goal. Several studies since his death have suggested that low body mass index and weight loss in middle age may be risk factors for ALS. If so, the calorie restriction that Walford thought was his ticket to longevity may actually have hastened his demise.

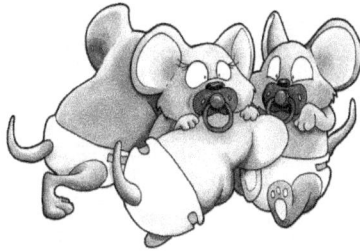

CALORIE RESTRICTION

NORMAL CALORIC INTAKE

DECREASED ACTIVITY OF
PI3K-AKT1-mTOR AXIS

INCREASED ACTIVITY OF PI3K-
AKT1-mTOR AXIS

MORE ENERGY INVESTED IN DNA
REPAIR AND CELL MAINTENANCE

MORE ENERGY INVESTED IN
CELL GROWTH

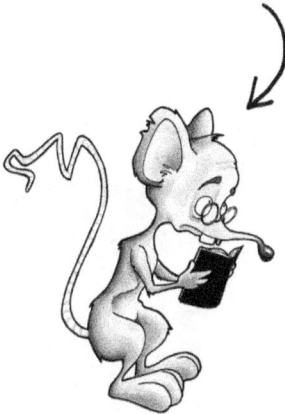

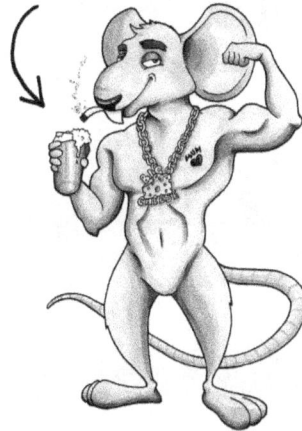

Lab mice subjected to calorie restriction live longer because they invest more energy into DNA repair and cell maintenance. However, they are frail, scrawny, and undersexed compared to their normally fed brethren. (Illustration by Ciaraíoch Art.)

PART TWO

THINGS TO AVOID

CHAPTER 10

So Salty

Moderate your salt intake by avoiding processed food and fast food, and eating potassium-rich fruits and vegetables.

By Hercules! The higher enjoyments of life could not exist without the use of salt.

—Pliny the Elder, *Natural History*

Our bad romance with sodium chloride goes back to the dawn of civilization. Humans harvested salt from mineral springs in the Alps as early as 5600 BCE. The earliest roads began as paths that animals made to get to salt licks. When Daniel Boone crossed the Cumberland Gap, he was just following a buffalo trail between Kentucky and the brackish swamps of Saltville, Virginia. The Romans only built cities near ready sources of salt, one of the few means of preserving food in the ancient world. Roman legions ran on sausages and hard cheese, both cured with salt. The word "salary" derives from the Latin *salarium*, an allowance paid to Roman officials to buy salt (that is, if they were worth their salt). Rock salt was used as currency in China and Ethiopia. Moorish traders crossed the Sahara with caravans of salt, and in Timbuktu exchanged them for their weight in gold.

How much do we love salt? We love it to death, quite literally. An estimated 1.65 million people annually die from excess salt intake. How much sodium is too much? The US Department of Agriculture dietary guidelines recommend less than 2300 mg of sodium a day, about the amount in a teaspoon of regular table salt. The World Health Organization is stricter, setting a daily limit of 2000 mg of sodium. The scowling puritans at the American Heart Association think you should be happy with 1500 mg a day, and insinuate that if you weren't a self-indulgent wuss, you could get down to 500 mg daily, which is the bare minimum necessary for survival.

The average American consumes 3600 mg of sodium a day. This seems like a lot, but it's better than the glorious nation of Kazakhstan, which has an average daily sodium intake of 6000 mg, the highest in the world. The global average daily sodium consumption is 4000 mg. In fact, 99% of countries have typical salt intakes in violation of the World Health Organization standard.

So, we're all eating way too much sodium, and should get below 2000 mg a day, right? Surprisingly, whether or not we should reduce salt intake is less clear than you might think. There is one thing that everybody agrees on: very high levels of sodium ingestion are harmful. In one meta-analysis of 25 studies, people with a daily sodium intake greater than 4945 mg had a 16% higher overall risk of death. (This number is somewhat skewed, because people who ate this much salt tended to be sicker when the studies began.) In another study, sodium intakes over 7000 mg a day were associated with a 23% higher risk of heart attack, stroke, or death, even after adjusting for the worse baseline health of the high-sodium group.

On the flip side, the evidence of benefit for aggressive sodium restriction is scant. In fact, low levels of salt intake may actually *increase* the risk of death. In the PURE Study, which looked at health outcomes of over 100,000 people from 18 different countries, people with a daily sodium intake of less than 3000 mg per day had a 19% higher risk of death, heart attack, or stroke, compared to those with intakes between 4000 mg and 5000 mg. Similar results have been seen in other studies.

Why might the risk of death be elevated at both high and low levels of salt intake? For people with high blood pressure and high salt intake, cutting back on sodium should help. If you are hypertensive, reducing dietary salt drops systolic blood pressure (the top number) by 3-4 mmHg, and diastolic blood pressure (the bottom number) by 1-2 mmHg. So, if you start with a blood pressure of 150/88 mmHg, you might get it down to 146/86 mmHg by eating less salt. Hypertension leads to accelerated wear and tear on the blood vessels of the heart, brain, and kidneys, and is a major cause of preventable death. Even slight improvements in high blood pressure lengthen life span.

But sodium restriction may also be detrimental. Our cells only work properly within a narrow range of values for sodium, potassium, and other electrolytes. Because our tolerance for wild chemical swings is low, our bodies are extreme in their pursuit of moderation. If our organs lack access to salt, they unleash a SWAT team of hormones to restore order, including renin, angiotensin II, aldosterone, and adrenalin. These make arteries clamp down, force the kidneys to retain sodium, and pump up heart rate and blood pressure. As a side effect, the renin-angiotensin system also produces inflammation and free radicals. While this frantic activity keeps our blood pressure steady in the short term, it ages blood vessels and tissues in the long term.

Whether or not aggressive sodium restriction kills is still a matter of hot debate. The anti-salt faction have made several valiant attempts to explain away the excess deaths associated with low salt intake. Perhaps these patients already had heart disease or kidney failure, and were told by their doctors to cut back on salt. Or maybe they suffered from chronic illness, poverty, or depression, and had low salt intake due to poor appetite or lack of access to food. The abstainers also contend that the harmful activation of the renin-angiotensin system is only a temporary response to salt restriction.

The Institute of Medicine, in its 2013 attempt to make sense of this mess, threw up its hands, and concluded that the "existing evidence, however, does not support either a positive or negative effect of lowering sodium intake to <2300 mg/d in terms of cardiovascular risk or mortality in the general population."

There is another aspect to this briny conundrum: potassium. Most of the surplus sodium in our diet comes from processed foods and restaurant fare. Potassium, by contrast, comes from healthy sources: fruits, vegetables, nuts, dairy, and whole grains. Sodium intake raises blood pressure, while potassium lowers it. The PURE investigators found that the lowest risk of stroke, heart attack, and death was in people who consumed moderate amounts of sodium, between 3000 and 5000 mg daily, while simultaneously having high dietary potassium levels. Only 0.002% of people in the PURE Study followed the World Health Organization recommendations for high dietary potassium with less than 2000 mg of sodium per day, suggesting that this guideline is unrealistic.

High potassium intake seems to reduce the dangers of high salt intake. Conversely, skimpy dietary potassium seems to magnify the risks of excess sodium consumption. In NIPPON DATA80, a Japanese study that followed 9550 participants for 24 years, people with high salt intake and low potassium intake had a 27% increase in the risk of death, compared to people with high dietary potassium and low or moderate sodium intake.

A final point: it is sometimes suggested that gourmet salts are better for you, compared to regular table salt. This claim should be taken with a whopping grain of salt. Black mineral salt and pink Himalayan salt are simply plain old sodium chloride with colorful impurities. The only benefits of artisanal salts are snob appeal and the frisson of possible exposure to toxic heavy metals (and maybe a dash of marine microplastics, in the case of sea salts). So stick with regular table salt, which has added iodine to prevent thyroid goiters. Wasting your money on gourmet salt, and then getting an unsightly neck mass, would just be rubbing salt in your wounds.

CHAPTER 11

Red Meat Rhetoric

Red meat gets a lot of bad press, but processed red meat should get
most of the blame. Avoid processed red meats such as ham, bacon,
hot dogs, sausages, and deli meat.

In November 1939, Joseph Stalin invaded Finland. This should have been a romp for the Soviets. The Finns had little in the way of artillery, tanks, and air power, and they were outnumbered three-to-one. So they resorted to guerilla warfare. Their soldiers glided on skis through frozen bogs and forests, stalling the plodding Soviet advance with raids, ambushes, and Molotov cocktails. And while the Finns were well led, the Red Army had few veteran officers, as Stalin had murdered most of them in purges.

As the Finns were preparing to attack a village called Tolvajärvi, the Soviets had a surprise of their own. A Russian battalion stormed out of the woods, slammed into the Finnish flank, and scattered them. In a normal battle, this should have been decisive. But the Soviet troops found a field kitchen with steaming cauldrons of sausage soup waiting for them. Instead of pursuing the Finns, they settled down to eat. The Finns rallied, and counter-attacked with fixed bayonets and submachine guns. The Soviet battalion was wiped out. It was said that the Russian corpses had bits of sausage still frozen to their lips. This engagement is remembered today as the "Sausage War."

The Battle of Tolvajärvi was a humiliating defeat for Stalin. While the Russians eventually forced the Finns into an unfavorable peace, the damage had been done. Based on the poor Soviet showing against Finland, the German High Command fatally underestimated the Red Army. Hitler decided to invade the Soviet Union, leading to four years of carnage on the Eastern Front, and ultimately to the defeat of the Third Reich. Would Nazi Germany still exist today if a battalion of hungry Russians had resisted the fatal allure of red meat?

Humans as a species have a deep and abiding love of red meat. (In nutrition science, red meat refers to meat from mammals that is red when raw, such as beef, pork, and lamb. It is red because of its high content of myoglobin, an iron-rich protein in muscle that helps to transport oxygen.) Anthropologists have suggested that the evolution and growth of our big brains only became possible when we obtained a steady supply of nutrient-dense red meat from hunting. But even if we evolved to eat red meat, that doesn't necessarily mean that it makes for the healthiest diet today, now that we have an abundance of other choices.

As long ago as ancient Mesopotamia, it was known that meat could be preserved by smoking, fermentation, or curing it with salt and spices. This processed meat was not only tasty, it also staved off starvation in times of want. Modern processed meats include sausages, hot dogs, bacon, ham, and deli meats such as salami and pastrami. Unfortunately, there is a large body of evidence that processed red meat increases the risk of heart attacks, stroke, cancer, and overall mortality. The World Health Organization considers processed meat to be a Group 1 carcinogen, putting it in the same class with cigarettes and asbestos. To see why processed meat is so unhealthy, let's look at what goes into salami.

The major ingredient in salami is raw pork, mixed with minced fat, sugar, spices, and table salt (*salami* means salted). Salt draws water from the meat by osmosis and dries it, reducing the risk of bacterial spoilage. Sodium nitrate, sodium nitrite, or both are added to inhibit the growth of the bacterium that causes botulism. They also bind to the muscle protein myoglobin, turning the meat a brilliant red color. (Gunpowder, which contains saltpeter, or potassium nitrate, was used in wartime as an emergency preservative, when no other curing agents were available.) This gemish is squeezed into pig intestines, and hung up in a muggy room for three days. Humidity encourages the growth of lactobacillus, a bacteria that excretes acids and ferments the meat. These acids inhibit the growth of other bacteria. The salami is then coated in mold, which acts as a further barrier to bacteria, and hung up to dry in cool conditions.

Processed meats typically contain 400% more sodium than unprocessed meats. High salt intake leads to high blood pressure and stiff blood vessels. This alone probably explains much of the increased risk of heart attack and stroke associated with processed meats. Processed meats are also linked to type 2 diabetes and several cancers, with an especially robust association with colorectal cancer. Nitrates and nitrites are probably to blame. During cooking, these chemicals react with protein to form nitrosamines, which are carcinogenic, and probably also toxic to the insulin-producing cells of the pancreas.

There's evidence that nitrates are not good for your brain, either. Dried cured meats with nitrates, such as beef jerky, have been linked to manic episodes. (Spinach, radish, lettuce, and other vegetables naturally contain nitrates and nitrites, but these foods have a low protein content, and rarely lead to nitrosamine production. They also contain vitamin C, which blocks nitrosamine formation.)

There is an interesting piece of indirect evidence for the dangers of processed meats. In the early 20th century, stomach cancer was the most common cancer in the United States, but rates have declined steadily since then. One explanation is that the availability of iceboxes (and later, refrigerators) to store fresh meat reduced our reliance on carcinogenic cured and smoked meats. A similar phenomenon seems to be happening in China today, with gastric cancer rates falling as living standards are rising, and more people can afford refrigerators.

While it is pretty much a slam dunk that processed meat increases your risk of heart disease, cancer, and death, evidence for these dangers with unprocessed red meat are weak. The risks seem to be less than with processed meats, and in fact are not seen in all studies.

Although unprocessed red meat doesn't have added sodium or nitrates and nitrites, it does contain other possible culprits, such as saturated fats, heme iron, and L-carnitine. (These are found in processed red meat as well.) Saturated fats increase LDL, or so-called bad cholesterol. It was once thought that saturated fat intake was a major cause of atherosclerosis. This is more controversial than it used to be, and we'll examine the evidence in another chapter.

We have an uneasy relationship with iron. Too little, and you'll feel listless and dull. Too much, and you'll be percolating in free radicals. Heme iron is abundant in red meat, which contains ten times as much heme iron as white meat from chicken. This is great if you're anemic, as the iron in heme is readily absorbed. However, excess heme iron in your diet is associated with a higher risk of death from heart disease and cancer.

Red meat contains a lot of L-carnitine. (Carnitine comes from the Latin *carnus*, meaning flesh.) This chemical shuttles fatty acids into the mitochondria, like a stoker shoveling coal into a boiler. When we eat red meat, bacteria in our gut convert L-carnitine into trimethylamine (TMA), which is transformed by our livers into trimethylamine-N-oxide (TMAO). TMAO increases cholesterol deposits and inflammation in the walls of blood vessels. High levels of TMAO in the bloodstream heighten the risk of heart attack and stroke, and increase the risk of death by a whopping 63%. (By the way, L-carnitine is a popular supplement used in industrial quantities by some bodybuilders for its supposed fat-burning properties. This is a bad idea. Our livers make plenty of L-carnitine without any need for supplements. Moreover, too much L-carnitine will make you smell like a fish, before perhaps giving you a stroke or heart attack.)

Interestingly, American studies tend to show that unprocessed red meats are harmful, while European studies typically do not. This may be because Americans historically eat a *lot* of red meat (although they're eating less than they used to). As well, Americans are more partial to grilling and barbecuing. These high-temperature cooking methods create multiple carcinogens, such as polycyclic aromatic hydrocarbons. These compounds are also probably responsible for the cancer risks of smoked meat.

Large amounts of red meat may raise the risk of yet another medical condition. Diverticulitis, in which outpouchings in the large bowel become painfully inflamed, is traditionally associated with low-fiber Western diets. Recent studies suggest that unprocessed red meat may also increase the risk of diverticulitis by about 50%. Poultry and fish consumption do not seem to be associated with diverticulitis.

If you must eat red meat, eat fresh red meat, and trim away the fat. Minimize your intake of grilled and barbecued red meat. And try to avoid beef for the sake of the environment. Cattle use 28 times more land, consume 11 times more water, and give off five times more carbon emissions than other livestock. We may broil beef, but beef is also broiling us through climate change.

Why Does Nutrition Guidance Suck So Badly?

In 2013, Jonathan Schoenfeld, a Harvard oncologist, reviewed the nutritional science on the 50 most common cookbook ingredients. He found that studies by different researchers had shown wildly different results. Some claimed that tomatoes, potatoes, carrots, corn, cheese, onions, lemon, milk, butter, and eggs all caused cancer. Others claimed to have proven that these foods all prevented cancer. Which raises the question: why is nutrition science so muddled and confusing? The answer probably relates to how this sort of research is conducted.

The gold standard in medical research is the randomized controlled double-blind trial. In this type of experiment, large numbers of people are randomly assigned to receive either a drug or a placebo, and followed over time to assess outcomes. To prevent bias from creeping in, neither the patients nor the experimenters know whether they are getting the active drug or an identical-appearing dummy pill.

Unfortunately, nutritional versions of these studies are expensive, labor- intensive, and ethically sketchy. Instead, scientists may look at the effects of different diets on laboratory animals, which may differ from their effects on humans. If human experiments are done, they usually involve small numbers of people studied for brief periods of time.

Nutrition science leans heavily on what are called prospective cohort studies. In these studies, thousands of people are interviewed about their food intake, and then observed for years to see if they stay well, or develop health problems like heart attacks or cancer. This type of research is useful, but has limitations that may skew the results. For example, people often underestimate (or lie to themselves) about how much sweets, soda, and alcohol they consume. As well, it may be hard to unravel why certain foods are associated with bad outcomes. If people who eat more red meat have more heart attacks, is it because of the saturated fat? The plethora of salt added to processed meats like bacon and hot dogs? Is it iron, or toxic breakdown products made by gut bacteria? Or some combination of these?

Another problem with cohort studies is known as healthy and unhealthy consumer bias. For example, people who eat more saturated fats tend to differ from the health-conscious people who prefer polyunsaturated fats. Lovers of saturated fat exercise less, smoke more, and are prone to overeating and obesity. Researchers attempt to adjust for these confounding factors, but it is possible that saturated fats get a bum rap because people who eat a lot of them have poor health behaviors in general.

Another potential source of bias and confusion are studies funded by food industry groups. For example, you should be skeptical of research funded by the Hershey Company purporting to show that chocolate reduces obesity-related disease. (Yes, this was an actual study.)

CHAPTER 12

Anger Management

Temper tantrums and a bad attitude can kill you.

Dear Leader was not happy. In fact, Kim Jong-il, all-powerful dictator of North Korea, Father of the People, Sun of the Communist Future, and Ever-Victorious and Iron-Willed Commander, was thoroughly pissed.

Jong-il was a strange and vicious man who wore saggy safari suits, and sported the oversized aviator glasses and towering pompadour of his idol, Elvis Presley. Under his inept and savage rule, North Korea had become a poverty-stricken backwater. While he chugged $2000 bottles of Hennessy Paradis cognac, ordinary North Koreans starved. His temper was legendary. He was prone to fits of rage in which he hurled ashtrays at his cabinet ministers and ordered summary executions. He was also in lousy health. He was a chain smoker, and thought by Western intelligence to have had at least one, or possibly two strokes.

On December 17, 2011, Kim was informed that a massive hydroelectric dam then under construction had cracked, and was at risk of collapse. Although the dam was the centerpiece of an economic plan to bring North Korea into the modern era, it was a rush job, and corners had been cut. Jong-il lost it, and started screaming at the top of his lungs. He was surrounded by bunglers and dunces! Must he do everything himself? He would go to the dam at once, and punish the traitors with great severity! Heads would roll! But the Shining Star of

Paektu Mountain never made it to his crippled power plant. Rushing to board his private train, Kim Jong-il keeled over—and dropped dead.

A psychiatrist might have diagnosed Kim Jong-il with intermittent explosive disorder, the technical term for hitting the ceiling all the time. People with intermittent explosive disorder are a menace to society. They are more likely to engage in assault, road rage, and domestic abuse. They are also a danger to themselves.

When people go berserk, their risk of having a heart attack, stroke, ruptured aneurysm, or fatal arrhythmia goes up for the next two hours. Rage makes the heart pound and blood pressures shoot sky-high. Arteries may go into spasm. Cholesterol plaques may rupture, and clog blood vessels in the heart or brain.

Anger also increases levels of inflammation. Two inflammatory markers, C-reactive protein and interleukin-6, are significantly higher in the blood of those with intermittent explosive disorder. (High levels of these proteins increase the risk of premature aging and death. Interleukin-6 levels have a particular connection with senescence, the process whereby damaged, worn-out cells devote themselves to poisoning their neighbors.)

Even if you're not flipping your lid all the time, just being spiteful and shirty may hurt you. In a number of studies, cynical hostility, a state of pervasive anger and distrust, was associated with higher rates of hypertension, atherosclerosis, heart attacks, and all-cause mortality.

Some of the health risks of cynical hostility are behavior-related. The cynically hostile are more likely to use tobacco and alcohol, and be overweight and unfit. It's a little tough to sort out cause and effect here. Does being hooked on cigarettes and booze, or being obese and out of shape, make you more hostile? Or does being bitter and angry make you more likely to drink and smoke and overeat and not work out? Perhaps, as seems likely, it runs both ways. (People with cynical hostility are more prone to depression, which doesn't help either.)

If you suffer from angry outbursts or cynical hostility, counseling may improve your emotional regulation. Cognitive behavior therapy may identify destructive thoughts and behaviors, and replace them with better and more productive ones. Some therapists use behavior reversal. In this technique, you act out responses to everyday triggers that are effective and socially acceptable, and learn to avoid ones that are not, such as committing assault and battery at your kid's hockey game.

As we'll discuss later, regular churchgoing is associated with longer life. This may be driven by several factors, including decreased rage, as well as increased life satisfaction, better mood, greater hopefulness, and stronger social connections. Agnostics and atheists might derive similar benefits from meditation or volunteer work.

If you're not spiritual, civic-minded, or excited about psychotherapy, you might still benefit from exercise. In one study, men with explosive anger problems were exposed to photographs chosen to make them angry. The images produced the same feelings of fury, and the same brain activity consistent with strong emotion, whether or not they had just worked out. However, men who had exercised could better control their anger, and were protected against long-lasting angry moods.

CHAPTER 13

Filthie Smoake

Avoid smoke, especially cigarette smoke.

Who was the greatest mass murderer of all time? Hitler or Stalin? Maybe Mao Zedong or Genghis Khan? Those are the usual suspects. But how about James Buchanan Duke, the father of the American cigarette industry, who is at least partly responsible for the deaths of Humphrey Bogart, Audrey Hepburn, Walt Disney, and 100 million others?

When "Buck" Duke took over his dad's failing tobacco company in the 1880s, the American tobacco market was dominated by cigars, chew, and pipe tobacco. Cigarettes were a disreputable niche product favored by urban riffraff. Duke's genius was in realizing that the lowly cigarette business was a potential goldmine.

Nicotine is one of the most addictive of drugs, and cigarettes are perhaps the best way to get it into the bloodstream. Plants grown on the red clay soil of North Carolina produce a mellow leaf known as bright tobacco. When this leaf is flue-cured, or dried in special furnaces, its sugar content spikes up, making it even more palatable. Unlike harsher pipe and cigar smoke, the smoke from flue-cured bright tobacco can be inhaled deep into the lungs, producing a nicotine hit in the brain moments later.

Duke is remembered today as a philanthropist and the founder of Duke University. But in his amoral pursuit of profits, he was more like a Tobacco Road version of Pablo Escobar. He fired the women who hand-rolled his cigarettes, replaced them with cigarette-rolling machines, and flooded the market with cheap product. He started a long and shameful tradition of cigarette promotions targeted at kids, luring boys with collectible cards featuring baseball players, Civil War generals, and busty Victorian actresses. He drove some competitors out of business, and forced the rest to join his cartel, the American Tobacco Company. At the peak of its power, Duke's monopoly drove the price of tobacco crops so low that bankrupt farmers in Kentucky and Tennessee turned to mob violence, burning and dynamiting tobacco factories in what became known as the Black Patch Tobacco Wars.

Tobacco has been suspect for centuries. In 1604, King James I wrote *A Counterblaste to Tobacco*, ranting about "filthie smoake" which was "dangerous to the Lungs." Unfortunately, no one took James seriously, as he slobbered, bathed once a year, and was obsessed with witchcraft. Because damage from cigarette smoke builds up slowly, and as we didn't live that long until fairly recently, it took time to prove that smoking kills people. Hard evidence that smoking reduces life span did not emerge until 1938. We now know that smoking shortens life expectancy by an average of ten years.

When I see a new patient admitted to the hospital, it is usually easy for me to tell if he or she is a smoker. As we say on rounds, smokers appear older than their stated age. (A dramatic example is seen in the differential aging of identical twins, where one is a smoker and the other is not.) A burning cigarette unleashes a smorgasbord of carcinogens, including formaldehyde, carbon monoxide, nitrogen oxides, hydrogen cyanides, and ammonia. Every puff of cigarette smoke contains 10^{17} free radicals. (That's the number one, followed by 17 zeros.) These free radicals are a chemical wrecking ball. They damage DNA and proteins, promote inflammation, cause cancer, and raise the risk of stroke, heart attack, COPD, asthma, and diabetes. Instead of the glamorous life promised by the tobacco industry, cigarettes actually lead to premature aging, premature disability, and premature death.

Everyone knows that cigarette smoke is bad for you. What is less well known is that all smoke, even in small amounts, is also bad for you. Automotive exhaust and fumes from power plants and factories contain a variety of toxins. The pollutant which is most strongly associated with a higher risk of death is called $PM_{2.5}$. These are airborne bits of fine particulate matter less than 2.5 micrometers in diameter. These floating flecks are miniscule. For comparison, a human hair is 60 micrometers wide, and a grain of sand is about 90 micrometers across.

If you breathe in $PM_{2.5}$, this fine particulate matter is small enough that it doesn't lodge in your airways. Instead, it penetrates deep into the lungs, going all the way down into your alveoli, the tiny grape-like sacs where you absorb oxygen into the blood. Inhaled $PM_{2.5}$ are toxic sparks that set off inflammation in the lungs, which then spills over into the rest of the body. They also trigger the sympathetic system, raising levels of epinephrine, and making both the heart rate and blood pressure go up. The smallest of these smithereens, known as ultrafine particles, may get into the bloodstream, and travel to the brain and other organs. (Ultrafine particles might also get into the brain directly from your nose by hitching a ride along the olfactory nerve, the nerve that sends signals from smell receptors.)

$PM_{2.5}$ increases the risk for lung disease, such as asthma and COPD. And because they provoke inflammation and generate free radicals throughout the body, they damage other organs too. Exposure to $PM_{2.5}$ increases the risk of all-cause mortality, and is linked to higher rates of myocardial infarction, heart failure, stroke, diabetes mellitus, kidney disease, Alzheimer's disease, and Parkinson's disease. (E-cigarette users are exposed to a slew of $PM_{2.5}$, plus a lot of other chemicals that may damage the heart and lungs.)

If you want to live longer, it's a bad idea to live near gridlocked highways and congested streets, which are major sources of smoke-borne carcinogens. Living near a freeway, or in an urban area with a dense road network, is associated with a higher risk of non-accidental death, after adjusting for income and education. (In the United States, Black and Latino populations have more exposure to $PM_{2.5}$ than Whites, partly because many interstate highways were rammed through communities of color in the 1950s.) Accelerated aging from exhaust fumes has been found in traffic cops in Shanghai, who had significantly more inflammation and DNA damage in their systems compared to a control group of office workers. (Air pollution in some Chinese cities is so dreadful that it outweighs the health benefits of running and other outdoor exercise.)

Air quality is declining in the age of climate change. Hot stagnant air means that less pollution disperses from cities in the summer months. Droughts lead to wildfires, which flood the air with particulates. Dry weather also favors a buildup of $PM_{2.5}$, as rains help wash pollutants out of the air. Hotter temperatures increase ozone production. Ozone high up in the atmosphere is good, as it protects us from ultraviolet light. But at ground level, it irritates the lungs, and increases the risk of death from asthma and other causes. Ozone is also toxic to plants. It is estimated that ozone will reduce crop yields by 10% by 2050. Unchecked climate change means a bleak future of tainted air and blighted harvests.

If you live in a city, what sort of neighborhood is healthier? In general, avoid concrete canyons. Deep street valleys lined with high-rises may be poorly ventilated and trap pollutants. Greenery is good. Trees, bushes, and green walls and roofs remove pollutants from the air. Trees also break up air flow, and the turbulence that results sweeps away particulates. Areas near parkland and green space with low vehicle traffic are ideal.

There is real-world evidence that lower air pollution leads to better health. As a condition of hosting the 2008 Summer Olympic and Paralympic Games, China had to promise to cut air pollution. For two months, China took 1.5 million cars off the streets of Beijing, and limited factory operations and construction. As a result, $PM_{2.5}$ dropped by 27%. With cleaner air, Beijing residents had less inflammation in their blood, their blood pressures and heart rates went down, and the birth weights of their babies went up.

Studies have also shown that life span goes up when air quality improves. In 1967, workers at copper smelters in the United States went on a nationwide strike that lasted for nine months. This slashed particulate emissions by 60% in New Mexico, Arizona, Utah, and Nevada. Death rates in these states dropped 2.5% during the strike, compared to the years before and after. Similar declines in local mortality were seen after the closure of a steel mill in Utah and a ban on coal burning in Dublin.

There is no safe level of $PM_{2.5}$. Lowering current national standards for $PM_{2.5}$, tougher policing of existing standards, and reducing tailpipe emissions are all likely to save lives. To make cities healthier, we need more electrified cars and buses, and urban planning that puts public transit, walking, and biking first.

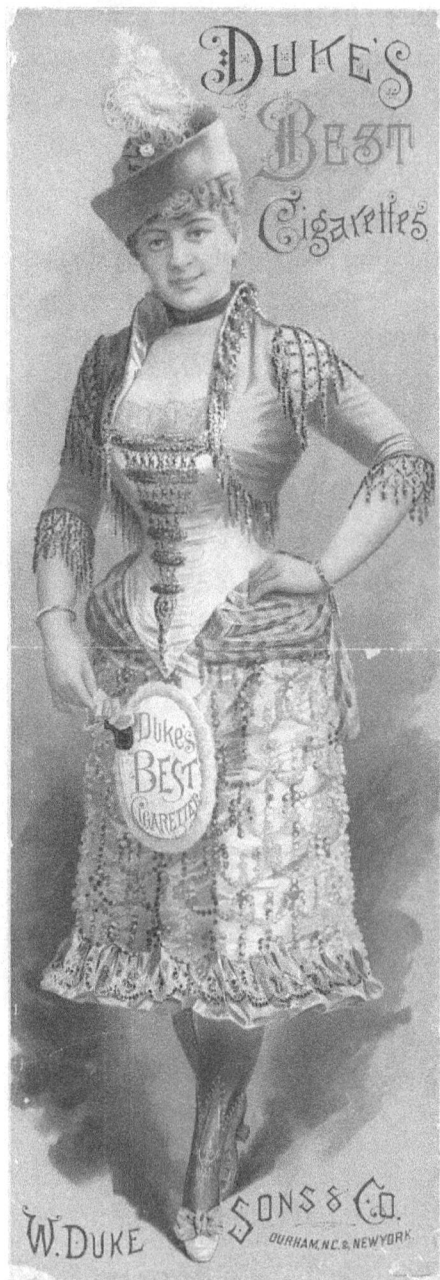

James "Buck" Duke began a long and shameful tradition of cigarette ads targeted at boys and young men, as in this slice of Victorian cheesecake (Library of Congress).

CHAPTER 14

Supplemental Discipline

Promiscuous use of dietary supplements may be associated with serious harm, including death.

The patient was a delightful 76-year-old woman who happened to be an alarming shade of DayGlo yellow. She had come to the hospital with jaundice, weight loss, and a tender swollen liver. Blood tests confirmed that her liver was indeed wildly out of whack. A CT scan of the abdomen was happily negative for cancer, and she had no gallstones on ultrasound. At the recommendation of a friend, she had recently started taking high doses of turmeric for arthritis. After she stopped turmeric, her abdominal pain eased and her appetite returned. In a month, her jaundice was gone, and her liver tests had gone back to normal.

Dietary supplements are big business. It's estimated that 38% of Americans take complementary and alternative medications, and the supplement market rakes in $40 billion a year in sales. Unfortunately, dietary supplements also lead to 23,000 emergency department visits and 2000 hospitalizations every year in the United States. Supplements are part of the Wild West of American medicine: a perilous and unpoliced frontier where profits come first, and safety and effectiveness are distant also-rans.

The supplement industry has long been coddled by Congress. In 1989, over 1500 Americans got muscle and nerve damage from a contaminated L-tryptophan supplement sold as a sleep aid, and 38 people died. After this catastrophe, the Food and Drug Administration cracked down on supplement manufacturers, who responded by sending an army of lobbyists to Washington. In 1994, the Dietary Supplement Health and Education Act (DSHEA) became law. This sweetheart deal allowed makers of supplements to sell them without proving that they work. In fact, they don't even need proof that their pills don't harm or kill people. They are only required to not claim to treat specific diseases. They get around this feeble restriction with impressive but vague declarations, such as that their products "support heart health" or "support brain health".

Because supplements are sold with limited, if any, official supervision and quality control, buyers need to be aware of potential harms. Some supplements have been found to contain lead, arsenic, mercury, and pesticide residues. The bacteria in some probiotic pills may spread genes for antibiotic resistance. Blue-green algae products, which supposedly prevent cancer, may contain cyanotoxins that lead to liver and nerve damage. And supplements touted as "natural" may actually be adulterated with prescription drugs and dangerous stimulants.

Of course, just because something is natural doesn't mean it's safe. Any natural product may have expected or unexpected harms. Plants naturally produce toxic chemicals to defend themselves from insects and animals that feed on them. Hemlock and cyanide are both 100% natural. Even when herbs are well-tolerated in small amounts, the higher doses in supplements might not be. Turmeric is a chemical smorgasbord, containing as many as 64 compounds with possible liver toxicity. The tiny amounts of these chemicals in curries are well-tolerated. However, the industrial quantities of turmeric that my patient was ingesting apparently led to serious trouble.

Even supplements that are beneficial in theory may not work in the real world. Beta-carotene is an antioxidant in colorful vegetables. Your body converts it to vitamin A, which is essential for your vision and your immune system. (During the Battle of Britain, patriotic Londoners were encouraged to eat carrots to improve their night vision during blackouts.) High blood levels of beta-carotene are associated with lower rates of heart attack, stroke, cancer, and death. It seemed like a slam-dunk that beta-carotene supplements would improve health and prolong life. But when beta-carotene supplements were studied in large clinical trials in smokers, it was found that treatment with beta-carotene actually *increased* the risk of lung cancer and death.

This unexpected and puzzling result caught researchers off-guard. It is unclear why beta-carotene was harmful in these studies. Did cigarette smoke interact with beta-carotene to make carcinogens? Do beta-carotenes have favorable effects at the small amounts in vegetables, but damaging ones at the large doses found in supplements? Are the benefits of dietary beta-carotene related to synergy with other micronutrients in fruits and vegetables? Or are people with high blood levels of beta-carotene healthier simply because they are eating less crappy processed food? These questions have yet to be definitively answered. In any case, you're better off getting your antioxidants from a diet rich in fruits, nuts, and vegetables, instead of lining the pockets of the supplement industry.

Toxicities of some common herbal medications and dietary supplements

Dietary supplement	Potential harms
Aloe vera	Colon cancer in mice (from drinking whole-leaf aloe extract; skin use safe)
Aristolochia (birthwort)	Renal failure, kidney tumors
Ashwagandha (Indian ginseng, winter cherry)	Used as a sleep aid, causes coma at high doses
Comfrey tea	Liver damage
Creosote bush (chaparral)	Liver failure
Maca (Peruvian ginseng)	Budd-Chiari syndrome (blood clots in the liver), endometriosis, breast cancer

Dietary supplement	Potential harms
Pennyroyal oil	Liver failure
Sassafras extract	Liver cancer and cirrhosis
Turmeric	Liver damage
Vinpocetin	Miscarriages
Athletic supplements	May be adulterated with: ■ anabolic steroids ■ ephedra (may cause high blood pressure, seizures, heart damage, and stroke) ■ high-dose caffeine
Calming agents	May be adulterated with antidepressant and antipsychotic drugs
Weight loss supplements	May be adulterated with: ■ sibutramine (linked to heart attacks and strokes) ■ ephedra ■ rimonabant (increases risk of depression and anxiety) ■ lorcaserin (may damage heart valves and cause hallucinations)

CHAPTER 15

Lost in the Supermarket

Avoid ultraprocessed foods.

And the peculiar evil is this, that the less money you have, the less inclined you feel to spend it on wholesome food.

—George Orwell, *The Road to Wigan Pier*

In 2019, doctors in England reported the case of a 17-year-old boy who had become blind due to a diet consisting solely of junk food. His height and weight were normal for age, and he did not appear to be obviously malnourished, despite having multiple vitamin deficiencies and low bone mineral density. He reported being unable to eat anything except French fries, white bread, sausage, processed ham, and Pringles, and was repulsed by the hearty texture of unprocessed food. The doctors restored his vitamin levels to normal, but his vision remained severely impaired.

Ultraprocessed foods now dominate the global food chain. In the United States, 59% of calories come from ultraprocessed food. Consumption of ultraprocessed food is high in all demographics in the United States, but is highest in young people, those living close to the poverty line, and those without college degrees. In Canada, a staggeringly unhealthy 62% of calories come from ultraprocessed food. (Perhaps our national obsession with Tim Hortons donuts is partly to blame.) Countries with strong regional cuisines are better off. In France, 36% of calories come from ultraprocessed food, and in Spain, only 24%. The United Kingdom, long maligned as a gastronomic dead zone, is a middling 53%.

Ultraprocessed foods are factory-made, and bear little or no resemblance to foodstuffs found in nature. They contain cheap industrial products such as high-fructose corn syrup or hydrogenated oils that are never used in home cooking. Chemical emulsifiers and thickeners keep them from getting runny or lumpy, and flavoring and dyes make them hyperpalatable, the culinary equivalent of crack cocaine.

Pringles are an excellent example of an ultraprocessed food. What exactly is a Pringle? The obvious answer is that it's a potato chip. But in 2009, Procter & Gamble, the corporate conglomerate who owned Pringles at the time, argued before a British court that their addictive concoction was *not* a potato chip. Potato chips, which are subject to value-added tax in the United Kingdom, are fried slices of potato. Procter & Gamble's lawyers argued that the Pringle lacked sufficient "potatoness" to qualify as a potato chip. Rather, the Pringle was an artificial Frankenchip, containing only 42% potato flour, mixed with rice flour, corn flour, vegetable fat, seasonings, emulsifiers, and a hefty dollop of salt. This caloric smack was molded into saddle shapes, flash fried, blow dried, and stacked and packed into cardboard syringes perfect for mainlining into our gullets. The Lord Justices were impressed by this argument, but not convinced, and told Procter & Gamble to pony up their $160 million tax bill from Her Majesty's Revenue.

Processing is not necessarily a bad thing. The oats in granola are edible because they have been steamed, rolled, and lightly toasted. Milk is pasteurized to kill *E. coli* and other nasty bacteria, olives are pressed for their oil, grapes dried to make raisins. But ultraprocessed foods have been altered in ways that make them fundamentally unhealthy. Processing pumps them full of sugar, fat, and sodium, and drains them of fiber, minerals, vitamins, and antioxidants. They are scientifically designed to be habit-forming. For example, Pringles contain the proportions of fat and carbs that have been shown to make lab rats gorge themselves the most. (Rats, like *Homo sapiens*, indulge in hedonic hyperphagia: eating for sensual reward, rather than from hunger.) From a neurologic perspective, being hooked on processed food is similar to drug addiction. In the brains of rats, junk food activates the same reward centers that are turned on by crystal meth.

In several large studies, a high intake of ultraprocessed food was associated with elevated rates of death. This increased risk seems to be at least 31%, and was as high as 62% in one study. This bump in all-cause mortality persisted even after adjusting for energy intake, smoking, physical activity, pre-existing medical conditions, and other confounders. Let's look at specific harms from ultraprocessed foods.

Glycemic index is a measure of how fast the sugars from a given food get into the bloodstream. Processing destroys the natural structure of foods. The more processed a food is, the more quickly absorbed are its carbohydrates. For example, the glycemic index of orange juice is higher than that of oranges. Ultraprocessed foods tend to have large amounts of added sugars, which makes their glycemic index even higher. (Refined or simple sugars have additional health harms, which we'll discuss more in the next chapter.)

Foods with a high glycemic index raise your blood sugars. In response, the beta cells of your pancreas get flustered, and release a wave of insulin to get things back to normal. Soon your blood sugars plummet, and all of a sudden you feel hungry again. This seems to be a major reason why people who eat a lot of ultraprocessed food have expanding waistlines.

A dramatic demonstration of the tendency of ultraprocessed foods to cause obesity was seen in a recent study at the National Institutes of Health in Bethesda, Maryland. Healthy adults were assigned to eat either a diet consisting of 84% ultraprocessed food, or one of mostly unprocessed or minimally processed food. Both groups received three meals a day that were equal in calories, and were also allowed to snack as much as they wanted. The subjects on the ultraprocessed food diet gained two pounds in two weeks, while those who ate unprocessed foods actually *lost* two pounds.

Having your blood sugars spike and crash like a demonic roller coaster has long-term health consequences. People who eat a lot of ultraprocessed foods may wear out their pancreatic beta cells, and are at high risk of getting type 2 diabetes. They are also more prone to get other pieces of the metabolic syndrome: high blood pressure, high cholesterol, high triglycerides, and increased waist circumference. Having all five components of the metabolic syndrome is associated with a 92% increase in all-cause mortality, compared to having none of them.

Trans fats have long been a major hazard of processed foods. Most trans fats in the twentieth-century American diet were artificially created by adding hydrogen to vegetable oils to make them semi-solid at room temperature. Trans fats are beloved by the food industry. They blend well, don't make foods greasy and oily, and are less prone to turn rancid. Unfortunately, they raise LDL cholesterol (bad cholesterol), damage blood vessels, and lead to heart attacks and strokes. Happily, they seem to be on the way out. The World Health Organization wants to eliminate trans fats from the human food chain by 2023. In the United States, the Food and Drug Administration has banned trans fats in processed food as of January 1, 2020. Tiny amounts of trans fats occur naturally in red meat and dairy, but these trans fats do not seem to be as unhealthy as the trans fats made from hydrogenated vegetable oils. (Pro-tip: avoid deep-fried foods from fast food joints! Trans fats may form spontaneously in superheated vegetable oils that have been sitting around in deep fryers.)

The gut microbiome. From a purely numerical perspective, we are more bacterial than human: our bodies contain more microbes than human cells. Most of these bacteria, collectively known as the microbiome, live within our gut. Diets poor in fiber, and rich in fat and sugar, change the balance of power in our intestines. Ultraprocessed food decreases the amount of beneficial bacteria in our bowels, and leads to a baleful bloom of bad bacteria. As a result, we may get irritation, inflammation, and leakiness of the gut lining, and be more likely to develop type 2 diabetes, non-alcoholic fatty liver disease, and irritable bowel syndrome. Low-fiber diets also promote obesity. Dietary fiber is fermented in our large bowel to produce short-chain fatty acids (SCFAs). These SCFAs bind to receptors in the gut, sending a satiety signal to the brain which curbs our appetites. Lack of dietary fiber means that we don't feel full, and are thus prone to overeat.

Carcinogens lurk in many ultraprocessed foods. Acrylamide is a particular worry. It is a chemical produced in starchy and sugary foods that have been baked or fried at very high temperatures. Foods with very high levels of acrylamide include French fries, potato chips, toasted sugary cereals, animal crackers, and gingerbread. Acrylamide is not unique to ultraprocessed foods. In general, the browner the food, the higher the acrylamide content. So beware of burnt toast, too.

Some preservatives may lead to the formation of carcinogens, such as nitrosoamines, which form when nitrites are added to processed meat. Packaging is another source of undesirable chemicals. Because ultraprocessed foods have a long shelf life, they are in prolonged contact with their plastic wrappers and containers. This not-fantastic plastic may leach bisphenol A (BPA) and phthalates. Exposure to these compounds may increase the risk of breast and prostate cancer, and also screw up gonadal development and function.

Sodium and potassium. Grinding and milling of grains such as oats, wheat, rice, and corn removes potassium, while promiscuous quantities of sodium are added as an all-purpose flavor enhancer. This combination of high sodium and low potassium in ultraprocessed food leads to high blood pressure, which in turn increases the risk of heart attack and stroke.

Phosphorus is an essential mineral, needed for both energy production and bone formation. In the human diet, it is found in the form of phosphates, in which the mineral is joined to oxygen. (This is good, because pure phosphorus has a nasty tendency to spontaneously combust.) A healthy diet contains moderate amounts of phosphate from meat, dairy, nuts, legumes, and grains. These phosphates are usually bound up in complex chemical compounds, and are therefore only about 50% absorbed. On the other hand, processed foods contain a glut of phosphates, added as preservatives, thickeners, and stabilizers. These phosphates are simple chemical salts, and thus are almost completely absorbed.

We've known for a long time that too much phosphorus can be deadly for people with chronic kidney disease. However, there is emerging evidence that excess phosphorus may also be dangerous for people with normal kidneys. In one recent study, people who took in more than 1400 mg per day of phosphorus, or twice the daily recommended amount, had a 123% increase in the risk of death from any cause. People who consume that much phosphate tend to overeat in general, but phosphates still seemed to be unhealthy when the researchers made adjustments for caloric intake.

Why would extra phosphorus be hazardous? A diet high in phosphorus could just mean that you're eating too much processed food, which is bad for other reasons. However, there are reasons to think that phosphorus excess is harmful on its own. Calcium and phosphates are the building blocks of bone. High phosphate in the blood leads to the formation of bony plaques in arteries, which increases the risk of heart attacks and strokes. The body also responds to extra phosphorus by raising levels of fibroblast growth factor-23 (FGF-23), which sends a signal to the kidneys to dump phosphates into the urine. Unfortunately, FGF-23 also has cardiac side effects, leading to an overgrowth of heart muscle that may eventually lead to heart failure.

So, for longer life, don't trust the process. In general, the more a food looks like something that was once alive, the better it is for you. Watch out for foods that masquerade as healthy choices, but are actually ultraprocessed, such as sweetened yogurt and sugary bran flake breakfast cereals. And support agricultural policies that make fresh, minimally processed foods affordable for as many kitchens as possible, while allowing farmers to make a decent living.

Glycemic indexes of selected foods. Foods with a high glycemic index lead to spikes in blood sugar and insulin levels, and tend to cause weight gain and metabolic syndrome.

Food	Glycemic index
Low glycemic index (≤55)	
Peanuts	14
Cashews	22
Kidney beans	28
Lentils	30
Whole milk	30
Apple (raw)	40
Orange	42
Grapes	46
Banana	50
Whole grain pasta, cooked *al dente*	50-55
Medium glycemic index (56-69)	
Orange juice from frozen concentrate (unsweetened)	57
Muesli	57
Whole grain bread	62
High glycemic index (≥ 70)	
White bread	70
Boiled white rice	73
Gatorade	78
Boiled potato	78
Doughnuts	80
Corn flakes	81

SOURCES: Foster-Powell K, Holt SH, Brand-Miller JC, Am J Clin Nutr 2002; 72:5-56; Atkinson FS, Foster-Powell K, Brand-Miller JC, Diabetes Care 2008; 31:2281-3; www.glycemicindex.com (University of Sydney)

CHAPTER 16

Children of the Corn

Avoid drinks and foods with added sugars.

Traditional Inuit cuisine puts the paleo diet to shame. Most of its calories come from fish, caribou, and the flesh and blubber of seals, narwhals, and whales, usually eaten raw, sometimes fermented and frozen. Before the twentieth century, cooking was not an option, given the lack of fuel in the high Arctic, and cooking would have destroyed the meat's vitamin C content in any case.

Carbohydrate sources in the traditional Inuit diet are scanty: seaweed scraped from rockfaces, roots and berries gathered in the short summers of the North, and the small amounts of starch in animal muscle, reindeer moss, and the partly-digested stomach contents of caribou, Arctic hare, and ptarmigan. Despite a diet that was considered barbaric and unbalanced, according to the conventional wisdom of the 1950s, Inuit were vigorous and free from heart disease, despite the ever-present risks of accidental death on the ice and the imported scourge of tuberculosis.

The Cold War transformed the Canadian Arctic and Alaska. The shortest route for Russian bombers and missiles to reach the United States was over the North Pole. To avert a Soviet first strike, American and Canadian military planners built a series of radar stations in the high Arctic, the Distant Early Warning Line.

With this influx of Western technology came a flood of Western food and the forced adoption of a Western lifestyle, with ruinous consequences. Protein and fat intake fell. Sugar, once a luxury, became an Inuit dietary staple. Otto Schaefer, a doctor with decades of experience in the Canadian Arctic, calculated that there was a 400% increase in refined sugar intake in one community from 1959 to 1967, based on his review of Hudson's Bay Company store records. Schaefer and others found that health problems that were once rare in Inuit communities were now common. The more sugary and Westernized the diet, the more likely Inuit were to have diabetes, obesity, high blood pressure, high cholesterol, heart disease, and diverticulitis.

Carbohydrates get a lot of bad press, some of it deserved. But there is a good reason that we love carbs so much. Glucose is the preferred fuel of our muscles and brain. In fact, outside of starvation conditions, glucose is the brain's only energy source. Our glucose stores are limited. We stockpile some in the liver and muscles, in a compact form called glycogen. These reserves are not quite enough to run a marathon, which is the main reason that marathon runners tend to hit the wall, or run out of energy, about 20 miles in. If need be, our bodies can make glucose from protein, and a little bit from fat, but these pathways are inefficient.

Because our brains rely on glucose, we have evolved to have a sweet tooth. Not all sugars are created equal, in terms of sweetness. Glucose, the major sugar in our diet, is moderately sweet. The carbs in wheat, rice, potatoes, and other starchy foodstuffs come in long strands of glucose, linked together like a chain of paper dolls. These elongated starches are rather bland, although digestive enzymes in saliva release some glucose from them, which is why they become sweet when we savor them for longer.

Sucrose, made from sugar cane or sugar beets, is familiar to us in its crystal form, as everyday table sugar. Sucrose is somewhat sweeter than glucose. It consists of two simple sugars joined together, glucose and fructose. As a standalone sugar, fructose is intensely sweet. In fact, it is sweeter than sucrose. Depending on your taste buds, you will perceive fructose to be two to three times sweeter than glucose.

Glucose and fructose are isomers. That is, they have the exact same chemical formula, but different arrangements of their atoms in space. In 1957, two Oklahoma biochemists discovered that a bacterial enzyme changed glucose into fructose in the test tube. A few years later, Japanese scientists scaled this reaction up for industrial mass production. Now any abundant source of boring old glucose, such as corn starch, could be transmuted into a sweet golden elixir. And so high-fructose corn syrup was born.

The new sweetener was less expensive than sucrose from sugar cane or beets, and it boosted sales of everything it was added to. High-fructose corn syrup wound up in a huge variety of processed foods: not just soft drinks, candy, and baked goods, but also supposedly healthier items, such as breakfast cereals, salad dressing, low-fat yogurt, and canned fruit. Although consumption has declined somewhat in recent years, the corn fields needed for the annual U.S. production of high-fructose corn syrup still cover an area the size of New Jersey. (Ironically, American taxpayers subsidize this overproduction of corn that makes them sick.)

Unfortunately, what was good for agribusiness was bad for public health. Fructose is not just a sexed-up version of glucose. The human body reacts differently to fructose than it does to glucose, resulting in metabolic mayhem. (Sucrose is sometimes marketed as being natural, and therefore healthier, than high-fructose corn syrup. This is not true, as both contain similar amounts of fructose.)

For comparison, let's look at glucose first. The physiology of glucose is a model of decorum. After a starchy meal, digested glucose enters the blood. The pancreas secretes insulin, and stimulates the liver, muscles, and fat cells to take the excess glucose out of circulation. The liver and muscle cells store it as glycogen, the fat cells convert it to fat. Fat cells then secrete a hormone called leptin, which suppresses the brain's appetite center to prevent overeating.

If glucose is polite and law-abiding, in metabolic terms, fructose is a scoundrel who jumps the line for the lifeboats when the ship hits an iceberg. Unlike glucose, which disperses through the body in an orderly fashion, all the fructose from a meal goes directly to the liver, and must be dealt with urgently, mainly by converting it to fat. This produces free radicals, inflammation, and fat buildup. Over time, non-alcoholic fatty liver disease may develop, with progression to cirrhosis.

The metabolic demands from fructose deplete the liver's short-term energy stores, which come in the form of a molecule called adenosine triphosphate (ATP). Loss of ATP and accumulation of fat make the liver resistant to the action of insulin. The liver also exports fat in the form of a particle called VLDL (very-low-density lipoprotein), which leads to obesity, and insulin resistance in muscle and other tissues. Because insulin is less effective, the pancreas must manufacture more. This added workload on the beta-cells of the pancreas leads to burnout, cell death, and type 2 diabetes.

Hypertension is more common in people who eat high-fructose diets. This may start at terrifyingly young ages. Teenagers who drink lots of soft drinks have higher blood pressures than their peers. Hypertension from fructose seems to involve multiple mechanisms. Used-up ATP from the liver breaks down to uric acid, which seeps out into the blood and interferes with blood vessel relaxation. High-fructose diets also lead to salt overload, inflammation, and high levels of the hormones angiotensin II and norepinephrine, all of which raise blood pressure.

Compared to glucose, fructose seems to cause more weight gain, perhaps because it leads to breakdowns in the mechanisms that normally prevent overeating. After fructose-rich meals, levels of ghrelin, an appetite-stimulating hormone, remain inappropriately high. Leptin, a hormone which decreases appetite, seems to be less effective in people who consume high-fructose diets. Magnetic resonance imaging (MRI) shows that glucose-rich drinks reduce blood flow to areas of the brain involved in appetite, while fructose loads do not. And unlike glucose, fructose activates brain regions involved in addiction. (Chocoholism may actually be a thing.)

Why does fructose wreak so much metabolic havoc, compared to glucose? The answer may lie far back in human evolution. About 15 million years ago, our primate ancestors were living in what is now Europe, reliant on a diet high in fruit, when the climate started to chill, and winters grew harsher. A mutation in a gene called uricase led to higher levels of uric acid. This surge in uric acid upended the regulation of fructose metabolism, such that fructose was shunted into fat production. Bingeing on fruit in autumn enabled our simian forebears to build up a fatty layer, which improved survival in bitter winters. But now, in times of fructose excess, this mutation makes us prone to obesity, metabolic syndrome, and gout.

Should you avoid fructose altogether? Absolutely not! Fruits contain fructose, but in modest amounts, and a more slowly absorbed form than the fructose in ultraprocessed foods. And fruits have other beneficial components, such as fiber, vitamins, and antioxidants. But as a general rule, stay away from foods with oodles of sucrose or high-fructose corn syrup, such as candy, baked goods, and soft drinks. In fact, the best evidence for excess mortality from fructose comes from several recent cohort studies looking at the effects of sugary beverages, which provide megadoses of rapidly absorbed fructose.

In the REGARDS study, which looked at health outcomes in 30,000 mostly overweight and obese Americans, each daily serving of a 12-ounce sugary soft drink was associated with an 11% increase in all-cause mortality. Fruit juices were worse: a 24% increase in all-cause mortality was seen with every 12-ounce serving of fruit juice per day.

Similar results came from the Nurses' Health Study and the Health Professionals Follow-up Study, which together followed 110,000 health workers for 30 years or more. Compared to those who rarely drank sugar-sweetened beverages, those who drank two or more sodas, sports drinks, or fruit drinks a day had a 21% higher risk of death from any cause. Most excess deaths were from heart attack or stroke, but cancer deaths were also modestly increased.

In the European Prospective Investigation into Cancer and Nutrition (EPIC), the association of sweetened drinks with death was still present, but was not as strong as in the American studies. The EPIC investigators followed 452,000 older Europeans for an average of 16 years, and found that daily drinkers of two or more sugar-sweetened drinks had an 8% increase in mortality, compared to those with minimal consumption. Overall, there is pretty good evidence that sweetened drinks shorten lifespan. So instead of Mountain Dew, you should Mountain Don't. (Sorry.)

Glucose

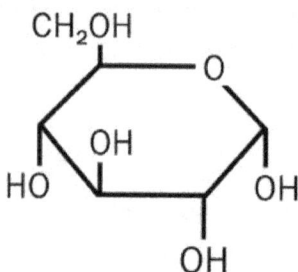

Fructose

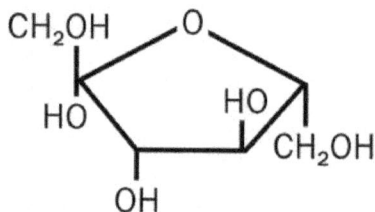

Although fructose and glucose have the same molecular formula, their structures and effects are markedly different. Fructose is two to three times sweeter than glucose. Unlike glucose, fructose is quickly converted to fat, fails to suppress appetite, and leads to obesity, insulin resistance, and hypertension.

What about added sugars in general? In 2016, a whopping 14.4% of the total daily calories in the average American diet came from added sugar in processed foods and drinks. (This actually represents a slight decline from 16.4% of total calories in 1999.) A high risk of cardiovascular death was seen in those with high added sugar intake in one large American cohort, the National Health and Nutrition Examination Survey (NHANES). Compared to people who took in less than 10% of their calories in the form of added sugars, those who took in more than 25% of calories from added sugars had a threefold increase in the risk of death from heart attack or stroke.

Results from two Swedish cohorts were similar, but also oddly different. As expected, Swedes with more than 20% of caloric intake from added sugars had a 30% higher risk of death, compared to those who took in 10% of calories in the form of added sugar. But those with fewer than 5% of calories from added sugars also had a slight, but significant, bump in mortality. The Swedish investigators were perplexed by this finding, which was seen in only one cohort. One possibility was that some who claimed to be avoiding added sugar may have been deluded or confused about their diet. Another explanation relates to the social role of sweets. In Sweden, as elsewhere, pastries and other treats are eaten at coffee breaks and other convivial occasions. The Swedes with very low sugar intake may have been socially isolated, which is a risk factor for mortality in many studies. In any case, an occasional dessert will not kill you.

CHAPTER 17

Hold My Beer

Stick to less than seven drinks per week, preferably red wine.

A drunkard is a dead man.

—William Butler Yeats, "A Drunken Man's Praise of Sobriety"

In the winter of 1722, the Venetian nobleman Caspar Lombria fell ill. Lombria was only 40 years old, and his physician, Giambattista Morgagni, considered him to have a robust constitution. Unfortunately, Lombria had a fatal overfondness for the pleasures of his native city. Venice in the 18th century was the carnal playground of Europe, Las Vegas in a lagoon. Lombria loved feasting, revelry, and lechery. Most of all, he loved his wine.

One drunken binge left Lombria in a particularly ropy condition. His belly swelled up, and he became twitchy and confused. Morgagni gave strict orders for Lombria's servants to keep the booze away from their master. Lombria sobered up, and his mind gradually cleared. But in the words of Morgagni, "being weary of the medical regimen (though it had been so beneficial to him), on the thirtieth day he relinquished it, and exposed himself to violent perturbation of mind, and great bodily exertion."

Lombria's besotted exploits led to a fatal relapse of alcoholic hepatitis. His belly was more swollen than ever, such that Morgagni felt fluid cascading from one side of the abdomen to the other when he pressed on it. Lombria's kidneys shut down, his delirium returned, and he "died like a suffocated person, with his face and shoulders very livid." When the body was opened for embalming, Morgagni saw that the liver was hard and shrunken and scarred, and the abdominal cavity was full of fetid yellow liquid. Lombria was probably the first case of alcoholic cirrhosis to be diagnosed at autopsy.

Before we get to the more vexed and interesting question of whether a moderate amount of alcohol is beneficial, let's establish that drinking too much is bad for you.

At a population level, even short-term reductions in alcohol use lead to longer lifespans, presumably by decreasing death rates among problem drinkers. In 1985, Mikhail Gorbachev cut alcohol production by 25% in the Soviet Union. Life expectancy rose, but government revenues fell. Gorbachev was forced to resume usual levels of alcohol sales in 1987. Alcohol-related deaths also fell during Prohibition in the United States, and in occupied Paris during World War II, when the Nazis stole vast amounts of Gallic wine for Teutonic consumption.

Alcohol kills 88,000 people per year in the United States. A little more than half of these fatalities are lethal misadventures: drunk driving deaths, suicides or murders committed under the influence, falls leading to blunt trauma, and other inebriated mishaps.

In the long run, alcohol leads to death from major medical problems. The most common of these is liver disease. Alcohol is broken down in the liver to acetaldehyde, which destroys liver tissue. Mitochondria damaged by acetaldehyde leak free radicals, starting a chain reaction of additional damage. The liver becomes fatty and inflamed. Liver cells die off and are replaced by scar tissue, and cirrhosis develops. Women are more prone to cirrhosis than men. A woman who has four drinks a day has twice the risk of cirrhosis of a man drinking the same amount.

Heavy drinking is associated with a higher risk of stroke, probably because drinkers are more likely to have high blood pressure. Alcohol also leads to heart damage. Heart failure and atrial fibrillation are both more common in long-term drinkers. (Binge drinking at Thanksgiving and Christmas is a well-known cause of atrial fibrillation, the phenomenon known as "holiday heart syndrome.")

Alcohol increases the risk of several cancers. Acetaldehyde, the toxic by-product of alcohol metabolism, is also a carcinogen. Heavy drinking is a robust risk factor for head and neck cancers, such as oral cancer and laryngeal cancer, especially in drinkers who also smoke. Alcohol is also linked to cancers of the esophagus and liver, and has a weaker association with breast and colon cancer.

Alcohol has two beneficial effects on metabolism. It leads to higher levels of HDL, the so-called good cholesterol. Drinkers have lower rates of heart attacks than the general population. I have seen alcoholics at autopsy with pristine coronary arteries, in striking contrast to their battered livers. Alcohol also seems to be associated with a lower risk of type 2 diabetes, probably by improving insulin sensitivity.

Current US recommendations are to limit alcohol consumption to 14 drinks a week for men, and seven drinks a week for women. (A drink is defined as a 12-ounce beer containing 5% alcohol, a 5-ounce glass of wine with 12% alcohol, or a 1.5-ounce shot of 40% alcohol.) But the studies that these guidelines are based on may have serious problems.

These recommendations come from studies in which the relationship between drinking and mortality is a J-shaped curve. That is, people who drink some alcohol seem to have a lower risk of death than those who don't drink at all. With higher amounts of alcohol, the risk of death rises, until it exceeds the risk of not drinking at all. However, the apparent benefit of moderate drinking may be an illusion, created by the fact that non-drinkers tend to be less healthy.

Compared to moderate drinkers, non-drinkers are more likely to be obese, diabetic, hypertensive, physically inactive, socially isolated, and have low education and income. Researchers attempt to adjust for these confounders, but it may be difficult to adjust for them completely.

In some studies, people who had a drink two or three times a year lived longer, compared to non-drinkers. As it is biologically impossible to have any meaningful health benefits from that miniscule amount of alcohol, this again suggests that non-drinkers as a group are fundamentally different from occasional drinkers.

Another explanation for the worse outcomes in non-drinkers is the "sick-quitter" theory. In many studies, people who used to drink, but don't drink anymore, are lumped in with never-drinkers. These studies may therefore be biased because these former drinkers could already have alcoholic liver disease, or other serious alcohol-related health problems. This might explain why a 2010 study by Jürgen Rehm and his colleagues at the University of Toronto had the bizarre finding that occasional drinkers had a lower risk of cirrhosis, compared to non-drinkers.

Finally, some supposed non-drinkers in these studies may be straight-up lying. There is no subject on which patients delude themselves and others with greater passion and conviction than alcohol consumption. For example, I once cared for a Yankee dowager with delirium tremens who adamantly denied drinking, even after her daughter found boxes and boxes of empty sherry bottles in her Back Bay condominium.

Shame and denial may extend to family members as well. As a student, I saw a 31-year-old man with a mysterious case of cirrhosis that baffled all our attempts at diagnosis. His wife, parents, and siblings all backed up his vehement assertions that his lips never touched liquor, until a cousin showed up from out of town, and casually let slip that the patient had been drinking a quart of Johnny Walker a day since turning 16.

Patient underestimation of alcohol use is widespread, and has been measured in many studies. If you compare population surveys on drinking to actual sales figures for alcohol, people underreport their intake by 50%, on average. (A possible consequence of this underreporting is that cohort studies may exaggerate the ill effects of moderate alcohol consumption, because some of the supposed moderate drinkers may actually be heavy drinkers.)

In any case, when minimal drinkers are used as the comparison group, rather than non-drinkers, there is evidence of harm at the current recommended levels of alcohol consumption. In a 2018 *Lancet* study of nearly 600,000 drinkers, all-cause mortality was lowest in those who had seven drinks or less per week. The authors projected substantial decreases in life expectancy at 40 years for those who drank more than this. Those who had 8 to 14 drinks a week could expect to lose six months, those who had 15 to 25 drinks per week would lose one to two years, and those who had 26 drinks or more a week would lose 4 to 5 years of life expectancy.

Another 2018 study, published in *PLOS Medicine*, suggested that the sweet spot for alcohol consumption may be even lower. In this cohort, the lowest all-cause mortality was seen in lifetime light alcohol drinkers, those who had 1 to 3 drinks per week.

Are some alcoholic beverages healthier than others? Overall, wine seems to be safer than beer, with hard liquor a distant third. All-cause mortality is lower in wine drinkers than in those who prefer beer and liquor. Wine is also associated with a lower risk of type 2 diabetes than beer or spirits. Beer and wine seem to provide similar protection against heart attacks, while hard liquor provides none.

Confounders could explain away some of the advantages of wine drinking. Compared to drinkers of beer and spirits, oenophiles have better health habits and higher socioeconomic status, and are less likely to smoke. And drinkers of distilled spirits are more likely to binge drink, which is dangerous because it quickly overwhelms the body's ability to detoxify alcohol. Habitual binge drinkers have a doubled risk of death, and also fail to enjoy the benefits of moderate drinking, such as a lower risk of heart attacks.

Is there any difference between red versus white wine? In the CASCADE study, Israeli researchers recruited 224 non-drinkers with type 2 diabetes, and assigned them to drink either a glass of red wine, dry white wine, or mineral water with dinner (the wine was provided for free). At the end of two years, the red wine group had significantly higher levels of HDL, or good cholesterol, compared to the mineral water group. Cholesterol levels were unchanged in the white wine group. The reason for superior metabolic effects of red wine are unclear. The red and white wines had similar amounts of calories

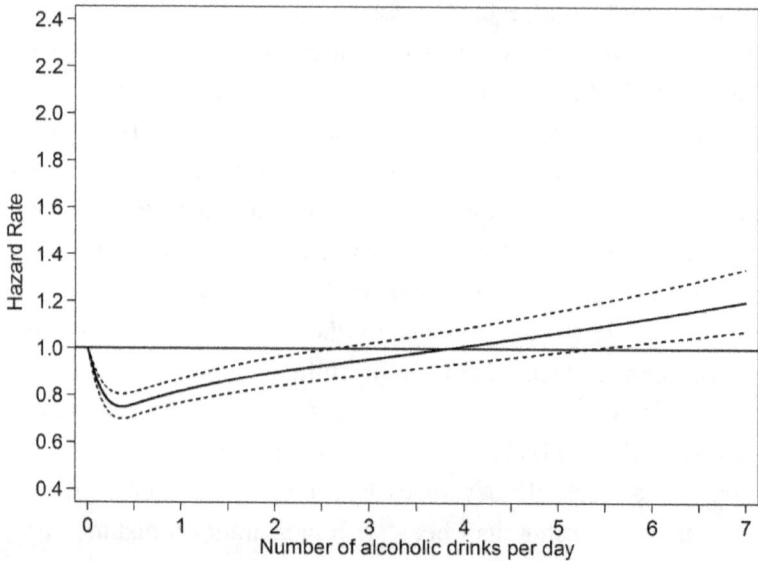

The relationship between alcohol and mortality in this study is a J-shaped curve (actually, probably more like a checkmark or a Nike swoosh), showing highest survival with modest levels of alcohol consumption. Other studies suggest this may be inaccurate, due to the inclusion of sobered-up heavy drinkers in the non-drinker category. Hazard ratios less than 1 means better survival, hazard ratios greater than 1 means higher risk of death. Dashed lines show the 95% confidence intervals. From Kunzmann et al, PLoS Medicine, 2018.

___

and alcohol. However, levels of polyphenol antioxidants, including the supposed longevity booster resveratrol, were seven times higher in the red wine.

A final caveat: as you might expect, a family history of alcohol use disorder confers a higher risk of problem drinking. If your family history, like mine, is a Hibernian black hole of drink, depression, and premature death, or if you've had issues of your own with drinking, you might do best to forego alcohol altogether.

CHAPTER 18

Trigger Warning

Avoid having a firearm in your home, especially a handgun.

Family and friends remembered Ryan Frazier as a kind, if troubled soul. While a student at the University of Vermont, he took a homeless man off the street, brought him to a restaurant, and gave the owner enough money to feed the man for the day. He doted on his toddler son, and won sales awards working for a wireless retailer, supporting not only his young family, but also his mother and two brothers. But by his junior year, he was sleep-deprived, burnt out, and battling depression. On November 13, 2008, Ryan stormed out of his apartment during an argument with his wife. The following morning, he was found dead in his car. He had gone to a nearby gas station, bought a handgun, and shot himself at an old railway depot. He was 21 years old.

The United States is currently in the grip of a suicide crisis. From 1999 to 2017, suicide rates climbed 33%, causing 14 deaths per 100,000 people in 2017. By comparison, the average annual suicide rate in Western Europe in 2016 was 9.6 deaths per 100,000. While life expectancy was rising in most Western nations, Americans were dying younger because of suicide and drug overdoses.

Talking heads waxing eloquent about America's suicide epidemic call these deaths of despair, and invoke economic anxiety, social isolation, substance use, declining church attendance, and the like. These may well be important, but there is another and more critical factor. Suicide attempts here are very often successful because America is awash in guns.

Just over half of suicide deaths in the United States involve a firearm. While only one-third of American households own guns, these households represent 60% of all suicide deaths. Teen suicide is also more common in gun-owning families. Within the United States, there are marked regional differences in suicide deaths. They are high in the West and the South, and low in the Northeast. The determining factor again appears to be firearm availability. Depression and suicidal thoughts are as common in the Northeast as elsewhere, but rates of gun ownership are lower, especially handguns. (Handguns account for most suicides by firearm in the United States.)

Many people believe that handguns save lives by protecting against home invaders. This is a myth. Living in a household with a firearm is more likely to result in your death, or the death of a family member. In a classic series of studies in the *New England Journal of Medicine*, Arthur Kellermann showed that having guns at home was associated with a fivefold increase in the risk of suicide, and a threefold increase in the risk that someone living in the house would be murdered. Out of all firearm deaths occurring in homes, 84% were suicides, 10% were murders of a spouse, relative, or friend by a resident of the home, and 3% were accidental deaths. (Because handguns purchased for home defense are often left loaded in child-accessible locations, such as nightstands, accidental child deaths are more common in gun-owning households.) Another 1.5% were justifiable homicides, involving an assailant known to the shooter. Only 0.5% of shootings involved strangers burglarizing the residence. So buying a handgun for self-defense is like entering a lottery in which there is a 2% chance of winning, and a 98% chance that you or a loved one winds up dead.

Kellermann concluded that rather than shadowy armed intruders, "the greatest threat to the lives of household members appears to come from within." The National Rifle Association, an organization which seems to consider handguns as a form of ectopic manhood, was so enraged at Kellermann's studies that they lobbied Congress to stop funding research into gun deaths, a ban which lasted from 1996 until 2019.

Suicide attempts may be planned or impulsive. Planned suicides typically involve people who are older, have a high burden of mental and physical illness, are tapped out financially, choose lethal methods, and take care not to be discovered. But most suicide attempts are impulsive, and involve younger people such as Ryan Frazier who are agitated after an interpersonal conflict. Long-term outcomes are surprisingly good in treated survivors of a suicide attempt. Only 7% complete suicide; 70% never attempt it again. Ryan's tragedy, and the tragedy of many others, is that the availability of a firearm turned an impetuous decision into an irrevocable act. I suspect that most people living under the same roof as a firearm have thought of suicide at least once; I know I have.

What strategies to prevent suicide are best supported by the medical literature? Drug treatment, and a therapeutic bond with a mental health clinician, may help control the ravages of major depression, bipolar disorder, and schizophrenia. Behavioral therapy may improve coping and problem solving skills. Social networks, spirituality, and having reasons to live protect against suicide. And limiting access to lethal means of suicide, such as guns, poisons, and overdose-prone drugs, also improves survival.

CHAPTER 19

Sitting Ducks

For longer life, get off your ass.

In the late 1940s, Britain was swept by a mysterious epidemic of sudden cardiac deaths. (In retrospect, this was probably due to the cheap cigarettes, fondly known as "gaspers," that flooded the market with the end of World War II.) A Scottish doctor in London named Jerry Morris wondered if these heart attacks were somehow work-related. When he looked at heart attack rates in transport workers, the data from London busmen was especially striking.

Bus drivers were twice as likely to drop dead from heart attacks as bus conductors. Drivers and conductors both came from the Cockney working class, and had similar lifestyles outside of work. But the drivers sat on their keesters all day long, while the conductors clambered up and down the stairs of their red double-decker buses collecting fares.

Morris then poured through the health records of employees of the Royal Mail, finding a similar relationship between heart health and on-the-job activity. Postmen who walked or cycled about delivering letters had low rates of heart attacks, compared to sedentary mail clerks and telegram operators. Morris then looked at national data on the death rates of workers in a wide variety of professions. He found that when he compared jobs paying similar salaries, heavy laborers had about half the risk of dying of heart attacks as those who worked at lighter occupations.

Morris became an early advocate of the health value of exercise. He quit smoking, and took up running, to the bemusement of his posh neighbors in Hampstead Heath, who thought he had lost his mind. Morris had the last laugh. He lived to be 99, and was still active in academia until a few weeks before his death.

Ordinary folks getting to sit in chairs is a relatively new phenomenon. In the Middle Ages, most people only sat on furniture at mealtimes on special occasions (*banquet* comes from the French word *banc*, a bench). The chairman was the guy at the meeting who was so important that he got his own chair, as opposed to the riffraff who squatted on the floor or leaned up against the walls. Now, many of us spend more of our waking hours sitting than not. But the chair, as it turns out, has been a public health disaster.

A meta-analysis of studies with data from nearly 600,000 adults found that the risk of premature death rises sharply at around seven hours of sitting per day, with a 34% increase in mortality in those who sit more than 10 hours a day. These studies had one major flaw: they used self-reported activity levels, which may not be reliable.

However, we do have higher-quality, objective data from the REGARDS study, which looked at risks for stroke in American adults. About 8000 people in this study agreed to wear an accelerometer, a device that records bodily motion, for one week. (Most smartphones and smartwatches contain accelerometers.) The participants, who had an average age of 64 years, were then followed for four years.

The accelerometers revealed that older Americans are very sedentary, being inactive for 77% of their waking time, or about 12 hours per day. As you'd expect, greater levels of activity were associated with better survival, and lower levels with a higher risk of death. The investigators were surprised to find that patterns of activity also mattered. Prolonged immobility was independently associated with a higher risk of death. People with frequent short bursts of activity had better survival, even if they were otherwise sedentary most of the time. The study authors suggested that moving around every 30 minutes might be the best strategy to offset the harms of sluggishness.

Two other studies with data from activity monitors also showed high rates of death in sedentary adults. In one of these, which used data from the National Health and Nutrition Examination Survey (NHANES), the least active 25% of participants had a six-fold higher risk of death than the most active 25%. These risks persisted even after adjusting for things like mobility, health status, and the protective effects of moderate-to-vigorous exercise.

How does physical inactivity shorten lifespan? Being a couch potato or a deskbound drudge has unfavorable effects on your metabolism. When muscles aren't moving, blood glucose levels rise. Conversely, levels of HDL (the good cholesterol) drop, because of the role of muscle in breaking down fatty acids. These changes increase the risk of diabetes and coronary disease.

A sedentary lifestyle also impacts mitochondrial health. The mitochondria, as you'll recall, are the power plants of the cell, where glucose is burned to produce energy. Exercise promotes mitochondrial biogenesis, boosting the size, number, and function of the mitochondria in muscle cells. On the other hand, mitochondria that are idle age more quickly. Sedentary older adults tend to have mitochondria that leak free radicals, leading to inflammation and DNA damage.

Finally, excess sitting is a risk factor for high blood pressure. In one study, every hour per day spent seated increased the chance of developing hypertension by 2%. Cell metabolism is sluggish in the seated position. As a result, the tiniest blood vessels, the capillaries, close up. Blood flow drops. Drag and friction along the walls of blood vessels, known as shear stress, also goes down. Shear stress sounds like a bad thing, but it is actually essential for healthy blood vessels. When the lining of the blood vessel senses shear stress, it sends a signal to the muscles in the artery to relax, which allows for greater blood flow. Over time, low shear stress leads to tight, stiff, hypertensive arteries. Sitting probably leads to high blood pressure by another mechanism. It kinks and bends leg arteries, and this mechanical obstruction also increases blood pressure.

Swollen legs from too much sitting also contributes to high

blood pressure. When you lie down at night, this fluid buildup re-enters the circulation. As a result, the soft tissues in the neck become engorged, increasing your risk of sleep apnea. These spells of obstructed breathing stress out the body, making your sympathetic nervous system pump out epinephrine, and your blood pressure skyrockets.

Long uninterrupted periods of sitting are especially bad for blood pressure. Taking breaks to stand and walk around lowered blood pressure in most studies. But a better strategy to combat hypertension if you work at a desk might be doing simple resistance exercises every half-hour or so.

One study compared whether walking or resistance exercise was more protective against hypertension from prolonged sitting in obese diabetic men. Light-intensity walking lowered systolic blood pressure (BP) by 14 mm Hg, and diastolic BP by 8 mm Hg. The resistance exercise group took three-minute breaks every 30 minutes to do sets of calf raises, half-squats, knee raises, and gluteal contractions. This group got better results, with a fall in systolic BP of 16 mm Hg, and diastolic BP of 10 mm Hg. (They probably also got some weird looks from passers-by, but whatever.)

If gluteal contractions in the workplace land you in trouble with human resources, try fidgeting instead. Fidgeting, or periodic leg movements, increases blood flow and shear stress in the popliteal arteries of the leg, which suggests that it might prevent the rise in blood pressure associated with chronic sitting. Standing probably helps as well. Compared to standing two or fewer hours per day, standing five to eight hours per day decreases the risk of death by 15%. Standing more than eight hours per day is even better, cutting the risk of death by 24%.

There is one sedentary activity that might be especially lethal: watching television. In one meta-analysis, 60 minutes of moderately vigorous physical activity per day seemed to cancel out the higher risk of death associated with excess sitting, except in those who watched a ton of TV.

In another study, doing literally anything else besides screen time was associated with a lower risk of death. A British cohort of 12,608 older men and women, who did not have a history of heart attack, stroke, or cancer at study entry, was followed for an average of seven years. After adjusting for physical activity and for cardiovascular risk factors, it was found that every hour of television watched per day was associated with a 6% higher risk of stroke or heart attack. Apparently, keeping up with the Kardashians can kill you.

Does science support the notion that television is a life-sucking force? Perhaps. People typically watch TV in the evening after supper, a poor time of day to be inactive. Sitting around after eating leads to higher spikes in blood glucose and cholesterol. (Ideally, you should go for a walk.) As well, people who watch television snack more, perhaps because they watch advertising that primes them to eat crappy food. Watching too much TV is also associated with social isolation and loneliness, both of which carry a higher risk of all-cause mortality. The idiot box is a paltry substitute for leisure time activities that are social, stimulating, and better for brain and body.

CHAPTER 20

So Lonesome I Could Die

Cultivate your social networks.

Without people you're nothing.

—Joe Strummer

In 1999, Dr. Gianni Pes told a French medical conference that he had found a region in the Italian island of Sardinia characterized by extraordinary longevity. In one secluded and clannish village, he had found seven centenarians in a population of 2,500. Not only were they still alive, some of these 90- and 100-year-olds still toiled in the midday sun, taking sheep to pasture in the rocky hills, before relaxing in the evening with a simple but hearty meal of minestrone and red wine.

The audience was unconvinced. There had been many tales before of remote rural utopias, where plain hard-working folk lived into outlandish old age, unspoiled by the moral and physical corruption of pampered city-dwellers, and they had all been bogus. In 1904, Nobel Prize-winning scientist Élie Metchnikoff hyped the health benefits of yogurt, claiming that its beneficial effects on the bowels was responsible for the purported longevity of Bulgarian peasants. A worldwide yogurt fad ensued. John Harvey Kellogg, the inventor of corn flakes and granola, became an advocate for yogurt enemas.

Unfortunately, Metchnikoff died a few years later after a series of heart attacks, in a temporary setback for Big Yogurt.

The mountains of the Caucasus were another supposed hotbed of longevity. In 1966, Soviet propagandists published an interview with Shirali Muslimov, a vigorous 160-year-old from Azerbaijan who had outlived several wives, ate apples from the orchard he had planted in middle age, and still rode on horseback. Skeptics uncharitably suggested that Muslimov had dodged the draft in his youth by stealing an old man's identity, a common ruse in Tsarist Russia. The isolated village of Vilcabamba, in the Ecuadorian Andes, was also said to contain an extraordinary number of centenarians. However, a careful review of birth and census records revealed that the oldsters were just grossly exaggerating their ages, in an apparent game of geriatric one-upmanship.

Despite his misgivings, Dr. Michel Poulian, a Belgian demographer who studied aging, was intrigued enough to visit Sardinia and dig into the official records of births and deaths. To his surprise, he was able to confirm that Pes had been correct: the number of centenarians in one part of the island was greatly in excess of expectation. On his map, he circled the area with an abundance of long-lived people in blue ink. And thus the concept of Blue Zones was born.

In addition to Sardinia, researchers have identified other hotspots for extreme longevity. These include the far-flung Japanese island of Okinawa, the Nicoya peninsula of Costa Rica, and the Greek island of Ikaria. These Blue Zones have many similarities.* Aside from an affluent vegan enclave of Seventh Day Adventists in Loma Linda, California, they have traditional lifestyles, verging on what some might consider backward, with modest but comfortable standards of living. Wealth and ostentation are unheard of. Hard physical labor is the norm, or at least was for the older generation. Diets are made up of whole foods, with high fiber content and low glycemic index. Most notable of all is the connectedness of their societies. Blue

---

* Longevity in the Blue Zones may also be related to happy quirks of genetics. For example, short stature, which is associated with longer lifespan, as we've seen, is common in both Okinawa and Sardinia.

Zone communities are cohesive, with robust ties of kinship, culture, and religion. Families are close-knit, with several generations often living in one household. Elders are not shunted aside into nursing homes, but are busy, engaged, and revered. It is almost impossible to be lonely in a Blue Zone.

In contrast to the Blue Zones, living alone, social isolation, and loneliness are now epidemic in many countries. These three things are not exactly the same. Social isolation is an objective lack of social contact, while loneliness is the subjective feeling of being alone. A person who is introverted may be socially isolated, yet not feel lonely. As you might expect, social isolation and loneliness are associated with depression, but they are also associated with medical problems. Older persons with social isolation are at high risk for malnutrition, falls, elder abuse, and dementia. Loneliness and social isolation increase the risk of coronary disease by 29% and stroke by 32%, with a similar rise in all-cause mortality.

How might loneliness and isolation lead to illness and death? We humans are social animals. From an evolutionary perspective, loneliness may be a hard-wired drive that makes us want to connect with friends and family for support, which in turn increases our odds of survival. Being socially connected may make us more resilient, lowering levels of stress hormones such as epinephrine and cortisol. During prolonged loneliness, these hormones may remain at high levels, increasing our risk of hypertension, diabetes, and other features of the metabolic syndrome. Loneliness may wear down the immune system. In one experiment, subjects with skimpy social networks who were exposed to cold viruses were more likely to get sick than those with a plethora of friends. Unrelieved stress may also lead to chronic inflammation, with high levels of the cytokine IL-6, which accelerates aging. During physiologic stress, less energy goes into cell maintenance and repair, which also contributes to premature aging.

Some observational data, but not all, support the chronic stress theory of loneliness and illness. There is another pathway by which social isolation may shorten lifespan: it leads to unhealthy lifestyles. People who are socially isolated are more likely to smoke, abuse alcohol, and eat unhealthy food. Social isolation also decreases physical activity. A study using wrist-mounted accelerometers to measure bodily movements for a week found that older adults who were socially isolated were more likely to be sedentary, even after adjusting the results for mobility limitations.

The American psychologist Harry Harlow is infamous for his horrifying experiments on baby rhesus monkeys. These studies, which would not meet current ethical standards for animal experimentation, may shed light on the corrosive effects of loneliness on individuals and social networks at large. Harlow first took infants from their mothers, and reared them in semi-isolation. They could see their peers in adjoining cages, but not directly interact with them. Some got surrogate mothers: wire cylinders with clownish heads that Harlow called "iron maidens". Later studies were even more sadistic. Infants were placed in isolation chambers that Harlow nicknamed "pits of despair". In these stainless-steel cells, they could not see humans or other monkeys, and were subjected to bright lights and a barrage of white noise. Loud sounds from the corridor outside made them freeze in fear. It was as if their childhoods had been replaced by a particularly bleak David Lynch film.

As you might expect, monkeys raised under these conditions became profoundly disturbed. They stared into space, paced restlessly about their cages, or grabbed their heads and rocked back and forth. The worst engaged in self-mutilating behavior, pinching a patch of skin on their chest hundreds of times a day, or biting and tearing at themselves. Attempts to introduce them into the company of other monkeys were at best dismal, at worst disastrous. Some cowered and refused to eat, becoming anorexic. Others were violent and filled with rage. All of them were sexually inept. Harlow abandoned his attempts at integrating them into monkey society when it became clear that they would all be driven off or killed.

Lonely humans may be a bit like Harlow's unfortunate monkeys. In one study, lonely people lose friends at a rapid rate, similar to how socialized monkeys drive away isolated, antisocial ones. Loneliness may even poison whole social networks, sweeping through them like a contagion. As their social ties erode, lonely people may transmit feelings of anger and despair to their few remaining friends, who in turn become lonely. As a result, the social fabric frays from the edges in, eventually becoming tattered and threadbare.

In a recent large meta-analysis, there were major gender differences in the risk of dying associated with loneliness. Lonely men had a 44% higher chance of dying, but lonely women had only a 26% increase in all-cause mortality.

Why might loneliness take a higher toll on men than on women? The reason seems to be a mix of bad behavior and bad biology. As all women know, men are lousy at asking for help, as well as being generally incapable of taking care of themselves. Studies show that men are less likely to acknowledge feeling lonely, less likely to seek care for mental health issues, and more likely to turn to alcohol in the face of depression and isolation.

Men and women also seem to have different endocrine reactions to stress. In men, the sympathetic nervous system is dominant, leading to the fight-or-flight response. The bodies of men under pressure churn out high levels of epinephrine and testosterone, making them prone to erupt with Rambo-style hostility and aggression, driving friends and family away. In women, this fight-or-flight response also kicks in, but it seems to be modified by the hormone oxytocin, such that women under stress are more likely than men to support others and seek out allies. This has been dubbed the tend-and-befriend response. (This may have evolved as a Mama Bear mechanism, prompting mothers to defend their young from danger, rather than flee.)

There are relatively few studies of interventions for lonely people. Older adults with social isolation may benefit from day programs, adult education, and exercise and dance classes. They may also have deficits in vision and hearing that affect their ability to interact socially, and may benefit from having these corrected. Older adults that are not computer savvy feel less lonely after coaching in internet use and video conferencing. Some universities are experimenting with intergenerational living, where students get free room and board in retirement facilities in exchange for helping older adults for about a dozen hours a week, often developing grandparent-like relationships in the process.

Pet ownership may make you less lonely, but some animals are more equal to this task than others. In one study, dog owners were less lonely than people without pets, in part because dog walking draws their owners into social contact. Cats, which are less attuned to human emotions than dogs, did not seem to provide the same degree of companionship. (In fact, cat owners were just as lonely as people without pets.)

In a small clinical trial, stressed and lonely adults who did mindfulness training were better able to deal with anxiety and distress that interfered with social engagement, and were more open and accepting of their emotions. At the end of the study, participants felt less lonely, and had more interactions with more people daily.

And there is also literature to suggest that people are less lonely when they do things that they consider to be meaningful and worthwhile. This includes walking or exercising, socializing with friends or family, doing cultural activities, going to social clubs or church, and volunteering. (Watching television tended to make people feel lonelier.)

CHAPTER 21

The Rich Are Different

Don't be poor.

They have more money.

—Hemingway, "The Snows of Kilimanjaro"

Poverty entails fear, and stress, and sometimes depression; it means a thousand petty humiliations and hardships.

—J. K. Rowling

In the heart of London, there is a road called Whitehall that is the home for much of the British civil service. In the sixties and seventies, Dr. Michael Marmot and his colleagues looked at the rates of heart disease in these bureaucrats, who were at that time almost exclusively men. English officialdom, like the society it served, had a rigid class system. At the top were the administrators, also known as the mandarins. These men were usually graduates of the glittering colleges of Oxford and Cambridge, accustomed to rubbing elbows with peers of the realm and ministers of state. Next came the middle managers, the professional and executive classes. Below them were the clerks, and furthest down were the messengers and other menial workers.

At the time, conventional wisdom held that heart attacks were a disease of top men, high-flying type A personalities with the weight of the world on their shoulders. But in fact, when Marmot analyzed the data from the Whitehall study, he found exactly the opposite. The bottom grade were three times more likely to die from coronary thrombosis than the mandarins, who had the lowest risk. The higher the pay grade, the lower the risk of heart attack.

Delving further into the data, Marmot saw that the risk of death amongst the different grades was very similar to the risk of heart attacks. The messengers and laborers had a threefold higher risk of dying from any cause, compared to the mandarins, with higher pay grade again being protective.

Some of the health problems in the lower grades may have been related to lifestyle. Men further down the pecking order were more likely to smoke, drink too much, and eat sugary, low-fiber diets, and they were less likely to exercise. They also had higher blood pressures and blood sugars, and tended to be obese. But even after adjusting for these factors, Marmot found that about 60% of the elevated risk of heart attacks remained unexplained, and seemed to be related to wealth and status.

While money might not buy you love, many studies have confirmed that it certainly helps you to live longer. In 2016, two Harvard economists, Raj Chetty and David Cutler, found startling evidence of the strength of the association between wealth and survival in America. Using de-identified death certificates and income tax filings, they calculated that the gap in life expectancy at age 40 between the richest 1% and the poorest 1% of American men was 14.6 years. That is, a 40-year-old man in the bottom 1% of income lived, on average, to be 72.7 years old, while a 40-year-old man in the top 1% would live to be about 87.3 years old.

This relationship is close to a straight line, aside from a sharp drop-off in the bottom 2% of income. Above this, there is a steady gain in life expectancy of about nine months for every jump of five percentiles in household income. The graph looks similar for women,

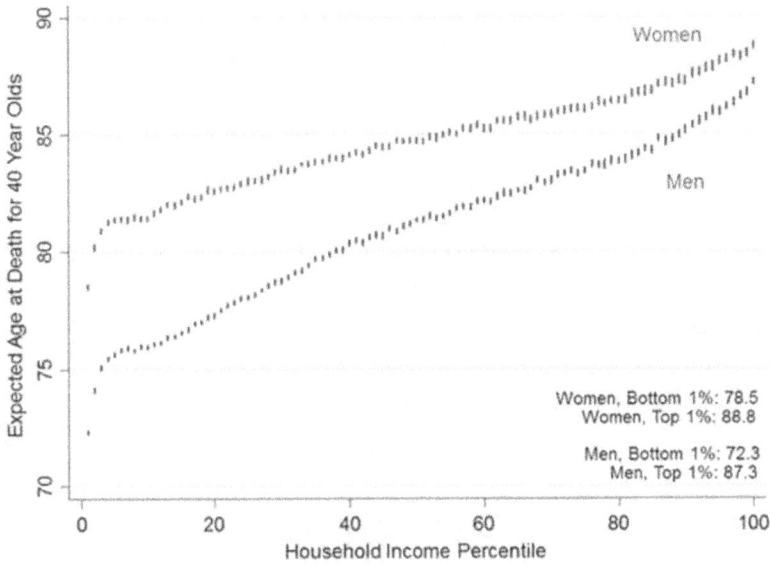

The life expectancy gap at age 40 between the poorest and richest American men is 15 years. Chetty and Cutler, JAMA 2016;315:1750-66 (image in the public domain).

although the lifespan gap between the top 1% and the bottom 1% of females is narrower, at only 10.1 years.

Chetty and Cutler found that the life span gap between rich and poor has widened in recent years. While life expectancy increased in the United States between 2001 and 2014, this growth was heavily skewed toward the top earners. Men and women in the wealthiest 5% gained another three years of life, while those in the bottom 5% got nothing at all.

Low-income Americans did worse in some parts of the country than others. They were most likely to die young in the midwestern Rust Belt, in states that voted for Mr. Trump in the 2016 presidential election. Paradoxically, low-income Americans lived longest in affluent cities with high costs of living, such as New York and San Francisco. This seemed to be related to lifestyle. Low-wage workers in these cities smoked less, exercised more, and were less likely to be obese. Chetty and Cutler speculated that in these cities, which have large numbers of college graduates, the healthy lifestyles of high-income workers rubbed off on lower income workers.

How does low status cause heart disease and shorten lifespan? We have a clue from studies done by Robert Sapolsky, a Stanford biologist who spent many years studying savanna baboons in Kenya. Baboon troops, like civil servants, have well-defined hierarchies. In baboons, this social pyramid is enforced by threats, intimidation, and physical assault. (Presumably, thuggery plays a lesser role in maintaining order among the bureaucrats of Whitehall.)

Sapolsky measured morning levels of the stress hormone cortisol in baboons, and correlated this to the baboon's position in the pecking order. (He accomplished this by knocking out the baboon with a tranquilizer dart, and taking a blood sample before the baboon woke up and tried to rip his face off.) High-status baboons had the lowest cortisol levels, while low-status baboons had the highest. Sapolsky also found that subordinate baboons had the lowest levels of HDL, or good cholesterol, while top baboons had the highest. British civil servants bear an uncanny resemblance to savanna baboons, at least in endocrine terms. Marmot and his colleagues found that low-grade employees in the Whitehall study also had lower HDL levels and larger spikes in morning cortisol, compared to high-status workers.

High cortisol and low HDL are bad for the heart. Low HDL promotes cholesterol build-up in blood vessels. High cortisol raises blood pressure and blood glucose, and leads to the apple-shaped fat build-up around the waist that is typical of the metabolic syndrome. Cortisol also siphons energy away from tissue repair and maintenance, and reduces antioxidant defenses against free radicals.

In experiments at the Wake Forest School of Medicine, Jay Kaplan and Stephen Manuck fed monkeys a diet loaded with lard and sugar, designed to clog up their coronaries. In most cases, the coronary arteries of subordinate monkeys had larger cholesterol plaques at autopsy. The one exception was an experiment in which Kaplan and Manuck scrambled power structures by throwing monkeys together from different colonies. In this war of all against all, in which the dominant monkeys had to start over and claw their way back up the food chain, high-status monkeys actually had worse-looking coronary arteries. (A plunge in status in humans also poses health risks. Job loss increases the risk of all-cause mortality by 63%. A wealth shock, or sudden drop in net worth, increases the risk of death by 50%, even if you still have plenty of money left over.)

Another factor in the reduced life span of people with low incomes seems to be an excess of epinephrine, also known as adrenaline. Epinephrine is a hormone that is released as part of the fight-or-flight response when we feel under threat. The immediate reaction to stress in the poor and the well-off is the same. The sympathetic nervous system revs up, the adrenal glands pump out epinephrine, and heart rate and blood pressure soar. But the recovery from stress looks very different in high- and low-status individuals.

Wealth is a wonderful buffer against the shocks of everyday life. To lack cash is to lack control and security. When your status is low, the stakes are always high, and the margin for error is miniscule. If you are rich, a traffic jam might make you late for your Pilates class; if you are poor, a traffic jam could cost you your job.

For the comfortable, when the moment of alarm is past, heart rate and blood pressure drop promptly. But for those who are just scraping by, heart rate and blood pressure take a lot longer to go back to normal. This faulty regulation leads to weatherbeaten blood vessels, and makes heart disease more likely down the road.

Looking at this data, you might conclude that biology is destiny, there will always be inequalities in health, and it is futile to try to set them right. But I think this would be wrong. Hopefully, human societies can escape the constraints of a despotic monkey colony.

For an alternative view, let's go to Scandinavia. Researchers in Norway replicated Chetty and Cutler's study of status and lifespan, using Norwegian tax and death registry data. Superficially, their results were similar to those of Chetty and Cutler. The difference in life expectancy between the bottom 1% and the top 1% in Norway was 13.8 years, almost identical to that in the United States. But the shape of the Norwegian curve looked very different. It overlapped the American curve at the bottom, between the 1st and 5th income percentiles.

But then it rose sharply between the 5th and 20th income percentiles, and stayed well above the American curve until the 80th income percentile, where the Norwegian and American curves met up again. So while the very poor and the very wealthy have similar life spans in Norway and the United States, low-income and middle-class Norwegians live much longer than their American counterparts. A 40-year-old Norwegian man at the 20th income percentile will live three years longer than his opposite number in America.

Norway and the United States both have advanced economies. Gross national income per capita in the two countries is nearly identical. So why do blue-collar and middle-class Norwegians live so much longer?

For one thing, there is less income inequality in Norway than in the United States. The top 1% of income earners in Norway pull down 8% of all income, while the top 1% in the U.S. takes home 20% of total income. Societies with more income inequality lack cohesion, and suffer from higher rates of violent crime, greater distrust, lower social mobility and educational attainment, and worse mental and physical health.

Work-life balance is also better in Norway. The average Norwegian works 37 hours per week, compared to the average American, who works 49 hours per week. The better status of Norwegian workers may relate to their high rates of union membership, which give them more control over wages and workplace conditions. Fifty-two percent of Norwegians belong to unions, compared to only 11% of American workers. And Norwegians, unlike Americans, are not crushed by debt from student loans or medical care. University tuition fees in Norway are minimal. While Norwegians do pay modest deductibles for health care, expenses over a certain threshold are free.

The dismal, and declining, life expectancy of the average American, relative to citizens of other developed countries, ought to be a national scandal. However, while the average Norwegian lives about four years longer than the average American, the poorest Norwegians and the poorest Americans have comparably short life spans. This suggests that poverty may trap people in a vicious circle of poor health. To steal the old joke about real estate, there are three reasons why: location, location, location.

The neighborhood that you grew up in may be as important as your paycheck in determining your life expectancy. Dr. James Cheshire of University College London found that the station on the London Underground nearest your birth home was a strong predictor of lifespan. For example, if you grew up near the tube stop of Hyde Park Corner, in the tony environs of Belgravia and Mayfair, you can expect to live to the ripe old age of 89 years. Four miles downriver, you will find Whitechapel station, in the East End. While no longer the ghastly slum stalked by Jack the Ripper, Whitechapel is still deprived relative to other parts of London. If you were born here, you will only live about 78 years.

In the United States, the health divide between rich and poor districts is wider still. In Chicago's North Side enclave of Streeterville, which extends from the Magnificent Mile to the shores of Lake Michigan, life expectancy is 90 years. But in Englewood, on the South Side, where eruptions of gunfire make people afraid to venture outside, life expectancy is only 60 years.

Unsafe streets are not the only barrier to health in poor neighborhoods. They have worse air quality. They are food deserts, with a paucity of fresh produce, and a glut of stores that sell processed food, liquor, and tobacco. Run-down housing is hazardous to your health. Mold or vermin in your tenement may trigger your asthma, or the peeling paint in your dilapidated walkup could give you lead poisoning. Stressed-out people in overcrowded households are also vulnerable to infections. People living in large households and crowded apartments had higher mortality rates in the first wave of COVID-19 pandemic.

Poverty undermines health early in life. There is an epidemic of asthma in children in deprived neighborhoods in the United States. Poor kids eat diets that are high in calories and low in nutrients, explaining why they are often both short and obese. Young people in poor neighborhoods are more likely to grow up to be adults with mental illness and substance abuse problems.

Childhood poverty embeds itself in the blood. Adults who grew up in deprived conditions have elevated blood levels of the stress hormone cortisol, C-reactive protein, a measure of inflammation, low-density lipoprotein (bad cholesterol), and glycosylated hemoglobin, an indicator of blood sugar control. These biomarkers indicate a high risk of premature aging.

The stress of poverty can also be measured in terms of DNA damage. In one study, middle-aged adults in highly deprived neighborhoods had lost an average of 95 base pairs of DNA from the ends of their telomeres, which is about equal to 7.5 years of premature aging. This relationship was stronger in men than in women, perhaps another indication of the greater biologic resiliency of women. A study in Belgian newborns suggests that differences in telomere length between the offspring of rich and poor parents may even be detectable at birth. (Racism is another stressor that may lead to tattered telomeres. In the CARDIA study, African Americans with more intense exposure to racism had faster telomere loss over a ten-year period of follow-up.)

Prolonged exposure to high levels of stress hormones warps the workings of the human brain. They disable the frontal lobes, which help plan for the future. They make the amygdala hyperactive, leading to excess anxiety and aggression. They destabilize the mesolimbic circuits, which are involved in motivation and reward. And they screw up the hippocampus, which is crucial for memory. The net result is that people under chronic stress are impulsive, react to unfamiliar situations with fear and rage, are prone to depression and addiction, and fail to learn from their mistakes. All these things make it that much harder to escape the trap of poverty.

In 1976, Dr. Thomas McKeown pointed out that the death rate from tuberculosis in England and Wales fell 90% from 1838 to 1948. This was a little awkward for the medical profession, as the first highly effective drugs for tuberculosis were not available until 1948. Before then, the treatment of tuberculosis was limited to cod liver oil and surgical procedures to collapse the infected lung. McKeown reasoned that most of the decline in tuberculosis was due to higher living standards, rather than medical care.

According to Michael Marmot, "Health is determined not so much by what doctors do for patients, but by arrangements in society." This may be overstated, but not by much. By Dr. John Bunker's estimate, half of the eight-year gain in life expectancy between 1950 and 1995 was due to medical advances, with the rest coming from social gains, such as higher living standards, healthier diets and lifestyles, safer workplaces and transport, and a more educated populace. In a study by Wim van den Heuvel and Marinela Olaroiu, looking at 31 European economies, national spending on social protection was a better predictor of life expectancy than health care spending.

Compared to other countries, the United States spends a great deal of money treating people who have already become sick, while making lesser investments in social programs. The net result is that Americans have mediocre lifespans and short healthspans. (That is, Americans tend to develop a high burden of chronic disease and disability at relatively young ages.)

In 1999, the Chief Medical Officer for the United Kingdom, Sir Liam Donaldson, perhaps inspired by David Letterman, produced a list of his top ten health tips. These were well-meaning, but somewhat divorced from the everyday lives of some of the people they were intended to help. Dr. David Gordon, Director of the Bristol Poverty Institute, produced a bitter parody, with the leading recommendation being: "Don't be poor. If you are poor, try not to be poor for too long."

The sad reality is that much health advice, such as that contained in this book, is of little value to people with low incomes. It is useless for me to tell a man of limited means to pick a stress-free time in his life to quit smoking, if he never has any stress-free time. (Low-income people try to quit smoking more often than high-income people, but are less successful.) It is foolish for me to tell a patient to take a walk every day if she is too frightened to leave her apartment because of shootings in her neighborhood. It is not helpful for me to advise my patient with asthma to avoid exposure to irritating chemicals, if she has to work a second job as a cleaner in an office tower to pay for her daughter's community college tuition. For many patients, poverty is the reason for their poor health, not a lack of knowledge, or a lack of willpower.

What sort of things actually help to improve the health of the poorest people? Dr. Marmot has suggested six steps to narrow the health gap between rich and poor. Every child should be given the best start in life, by making sure mothers get prenatal care, by reducing child poverty, and by increasing programs for early childhood development. Societies should invest in schools in deprived neighborhoods, and make post-secondary education more affordable. The status of workers should be improved with higher minimum wages, and job training to offset the impact of automation. Everyone should have healthy housing, and the minimum income necessary for health (a universal basic income). Finally, Marmot recommends a proactive health system that aims to prevent disease and improve population health, rather than merely react to health problems once they develop.

	The Chief Medical Officer's Ten Tips for Better Health	Alternative Health Tips from Dr. David Gordon
1	Don't smoke. If you can, stop. If you can't, cut down.	Don't be poor. If you are poor, try not to be poor for too long.
2	Follow a balanced diet with plenty of fruit and vegetables.	Don't live in a deprived area. If you do, move.
3	Keep physically active.	Don't be disabled or have a disabled child.
4	Manage stress by, for example, talking things through and making time to relax.	Don't work in a stressful low-paid manual job.
5	If you drink alcohol, do so in moderation.	Don't live in damp, low quality housing or be homeless.

	The Chief Medical Officer's Ten Tips for Better Health	**Alternative Health Tips from Dr. David Gordon**
6	Cover up in the sun, and protect children from sunburn.	Be able to afford to pay for social activities and annual holidays.
7	Practice safer sex.	Don't be a lone parent.
8	Take up cancer screening opportunities.	Claim all benefits to which you are entitled.
9	Be safe on the roads.	Be able to afford to own a car.
10	Learn the First Aid ABC: airways, breathing and circulation.	Use education as an opportunity to improve your socio-economic position.
	SOURCE: Department of Health, Saving Lives: Our Healthier Nation. London: The Stationery Office.	SOURCE: David Gordon, Townsend Centre for International Poverty Research, University of Bristol.

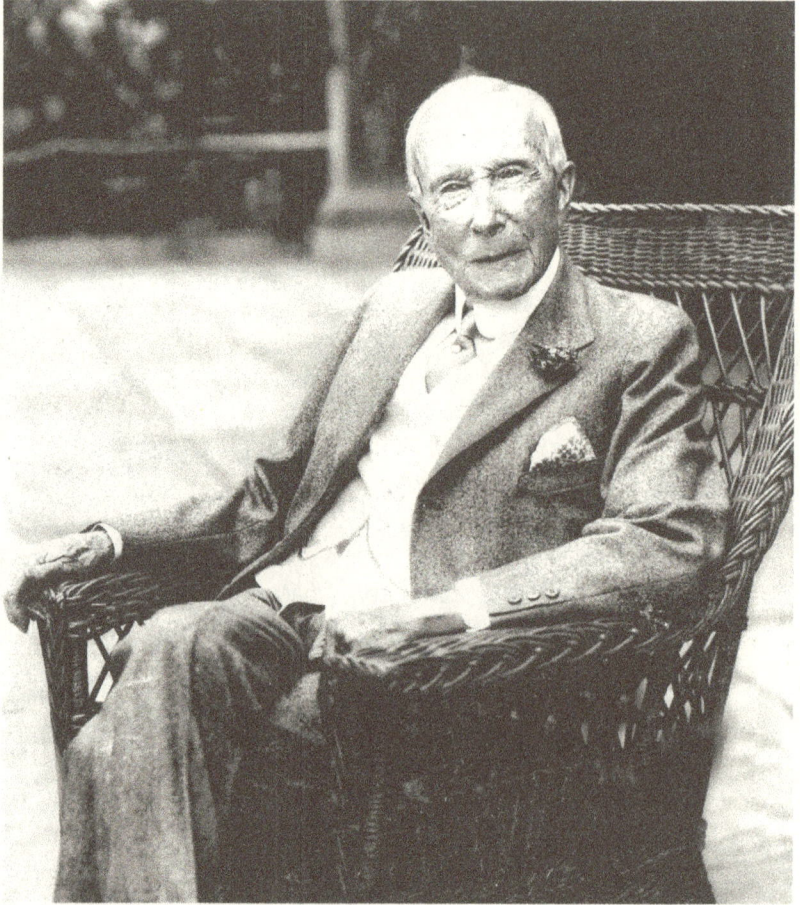

John D. Rockefeller, the richest American of his era and perhaps of all time, who lived to be 97. Rockefeller was a fitness buff and control freak who used his vast wealth to shape his society and his surroundings to suit his imperial whims. (There seems to be no truth to the story that the secret of his longevity was breast milk from a succession of Scottish wet nurses.) National Portrait Gallery.

PART THREE

THINGS TO DO

CHAPTER 22

Pressure Drop

Get your blood pressure under control.

The Reverend Stephen Hales became the perpetual curate of Teddington in 1709, and stayed in this post for the next 52 years. As Teddington was a sleepy English village of some 500 souls, his parish duties were light, giving Hales ample leisure to indulge his scientific curiosity.

At the time, some believed that the pumping of the heart drove the movements of the muscles. Hales was skeptical that arteries had enough hydraulic force to power the arms and legs. To disprove this, he performed a series of unsavory experiments in horses and dogs.

In the first of these, his assistants tied down a sick old mare. Hales inserted a brass tube into an artery in the mare's leg, and connected this tube to a nine-foot high glass cylinder. The column of blood in the glass cylinder rose to a height of eight feet and three inches above the level of the horse's heart. Hales had performed the first ever measurement of blood pressure. (We now measure blood pressure as the height of a column of mercury, rather than blood.)

Hales made several observations that are fundamental to our modern understanding of blood pressure. The column of equine blood rose and fell with each pulse. These swings correspond to systolic and diastolic blood pressure, or the top and bottom numbers of your blood pressure as measured at the doctor's office. Hales found that blood pressure rose with stress and pain. He also discovered that blood pressure could fall too low. With the evacuation of 14 quarts of blood, the column dropped to four feet high. The poor mare became clammy and cold, a victim of what we now call shock.

Hales' parishioners and friends, including the animal-loving poet Alexander Pope, deplored these gory studies as cruel and unbecoming of a man of the cloth. So the curious reverend turned to milder endeavors, such as measuring the force of sap in trees.

As patients proved as reluctant as old mares to have brass tubes stuck in their arteries, the study of blood pressure in humans stagnated until 1896, when the Italian physician Scipione Riva-Ricci invented the modern sphygmomanometer, with the now-familiar inflatable cuff wrapped around the upper arm. But American doctors were slow to adopt the newfangled gizmo. Many fretted that this intrusion of technology would ruin the doctor-patient relationship. Others clinicians scoffed at the new device, believing that they had near-mystical abilities to diagnose patients by feeling their pulses. This was, of course, a load of balderdash. But, like a lot of intellectual balderdash, it proved hard to kill.

Early evidence for the dangers of high blood pressure came from an unlikely source: American life insurance actuaries. By 1914, John Walton Fisher, medical director for the insurance behemoth Northwestern Mutual, refused to insure otherwise healthy applicants with systolic blood pressures over 160 mm Hg, as their risk of death was double that of applicants with normal blood pressures.

While insurers saw hypertension as a financial liability, physicians continued to regard it as a feature of normal aging, and failed to see that it sped up wear and tear on blood vessels, leading to critical damage to the brain, heart, and kidneys. The term *benign essential hypertension* was widely used, reflecting the wrongheaded belief that high blood pressure was both harmless and inevitable. Cardiologists such as Paul Dudley White, who attended President Eisenhower during his heart attack in office, thought that it was meddlesome to treat high blood pressure in patients who felt well. In the final years of his life, Franklin Delano Roosevelt's blood pressure regularly topped 200/100 mm Hg, and at the Yalta Conference, his blood pressure was as high as 260/150 mm Hg. FDR often appeared lost during the proceedings, which made extensive concessions to Stalin on the shape of postwar Europe. Two months later, Roosevelt died of a massive stroke at the age of 63.

Therapeutic nihilism was made easier by the lack of safe and effective therapies for high blood pressure. Potassium thiocyanate caused cyanide poisoning, reserpine led to suicidal depression, and sedatives such as bromides and barbiturates were prone to overdose. Until the 1960s, the gold standard of treatment for hypertension was weight loss, exercise, salt restriction, and stress reduction.

When better drugs became available, especially the thiazide diuretics, robust evidence in favor of treatment finally emerged. In a recent review of trials in patients 60 or older, antihypertensive treatment reduced the risk of death by 9%, the risk of heart attack by 22%, and the risk of stroke by 34%, compared to placebo or no treatment. There are not many good studies of high blood pressure in people aged 18 to 59 years old, but what data we have suggests that treatment cuts the risk of strokes in half.

One of the pivotal studies in the treatment of hypertension was the ALLHAT trial, published in 2002. This study enrolled over 30,000 participants, and compared three blood pressure-lowering drugs: chlorthalidone, lisinopril, and amlodipine. (One arm of the trial was stopped early, as the study drug, doxazosin, was found to be clearly inferior.) Chlorthalidone achieved the largest drop in systolic blood pressure (SBP), and amlodipine led to the greatest fall in diastolic blood pressure (DBP). Overall, chlorthalidone seemed to perform best. It was better at preventing heart attacks, strokes, and heart failure than lisinopril, and better than amlodipine at preventing heart failure.

Ideal blood pressure seems to be around 115/75 mm Hg. For every increase of 20/10 mm Hg above this baseline, there is a doubling of the risk of death from stroke and heart attacks. In addition to causing catastrophic clots and bleeds, high blood pressure may also damage small blood vessels in the brain. Brain MRIs in hypertensive patients often show silent strokes and brain shrinkage. Treating high blood pressure seems to reduce the risk of cognitive impairment and dementia. Controlling high blood pressure also reduces the risk of heart failure, atrial fibrillation, and chronic kidney disease.

High blood pressure has reached epidemic proportions, affecting 45% of American adults, and 72% over the age of 60. It seems the usual lifestyle suspects are to blame: too much dietary salt and fructose and too little physical activity. Fructose, found in many ultraprocessed foods in the form of high-fructose corn syrup, stimulates the kidneys to reabsorb sodium, rather than pee it out. Salt retention is worsened by the high sodium content of processed foods.

A toxic Western diet also tends to raise blood pressure by making blood vessels contract and tighten up. Weight gain from processed foods leads to high insulin levels. Too much insulin increases levels of endothelin-1 and thromboxane A2. These chemical messengers are vasoconstrictors, signaling the muscles lining the blood vessels to clamp down. To make matters worse, levels of nitric oxide, a chemical signal that relaxes blood vessels, are decreased by uric acid, which is a byproduct of fructose metabolism.

As ultraprocessed food is a major cause of hypertension, it should not be surprising that eating *whole foods* is associated with lower blood pressures. There is excellent evidence for the DASH diet for reducing blood pressure. The DASH diet is rich in fruits, vegetables, and whole grains, high in fiber, and low in sweets. Because of its whole food content, it also contains an abundance of potassium and is low in sodium, a pattern of mineral intake which is associated with better blood pressure control and vascular health. In clinical trials, the DASH diet was associated with an 11 mm Hg drop in SBP. (The DASH diet takes its name from the clinical trial that studied it, Dietary Approaches to Stop Hypertension.)

Other healthy lifestyle interventions reduce hypertension. For those who are overweight, *weight loss* will cause blood pressure to fall 1 mm Hg of SBP for every kilogram (2.2 lbs) that is shed. If you are a regular drinker, *reducing alcohol consumption* cuts SBP by about 4 mm Hg. Regular *aerobic exercise* drops SBP by 5-8 mm Hg. (The International Society of Hypertension guidelines suggest that *meditation and mindfulness practices* and *avoidance of air pollution* may also help reduce blood pressure.)

If you are taking antihypertensive medications, you should be aware of their side effects. Chlorthalidone lowers potassium levels, so it may need to be taken with potassium supplements. Kidney function may be affected by lisinopril and losartan. Both may cause cough as a nuisance side effect, especially lisinopril. Amlodipine may cause ankle swelling, especially at higher doses.

If your doctor wants to add a second medication to control your blood pressure, don't view this as a defeat. Most patients need two medications to optimize their blood pressure. If your blood pressure is hard to control, your doctor should consider checking for underlying causes. The most common of these is sleep apnea, in which the airway is blocked off by an excess of soft tissue in the back of the throat during sleep. This leads to recurrent nocturnal episodes in which breathing is obstructed, the body's stress response is activated, epinephrine is released, and blood pressure soars.

CHAPTER 23

The Weight

Maintain a healthy weight with physical activity and a diet
of whole foods.

What is the best build for longevity? Everyone agrees that obesity shortens your lifespan. However, there is still debate about whether the optimal physique is midway between bony and fat, or whether it skews more towards the skinny side. A vigorous advocate of the latter view was 1950s socialite Babe Paley, who is said to have coined the phrase, "You can never be too rich or too thin." Likewise, present-day fans of calorie restriction practice the gospel of semi-starvation for maximal lifespan. Lisa Walford, daughter of Roy Walford of Biosphere 2 fame, has driven her body mass index down to 17.

Body mass index (BMI) is your weight in kilograms, divided by the square of your height in meters. (If thinking about this makes your brain hurt, the Centers for Disease Control has an online BMI calculator, into which you can plug either kilograms and centimeters, or pounds and feet and inches.)

Normal BMI is between 18.5 and 24.9. A BMI under 18.5 is considered underweight. Some prominent examples: Kate Moss, who personified the heroin chic fashion aesthetic of the 1990s, had a BMI of 16. Aptly-named 1960s supermodel Twiggy had a BMI of 15. During his Thin White Duke phase, when he was consuming industrial quantities of cocaine, David Bowie's BMI fell as low as 14.

A BMI between 25 and 29.9 is overweight, while obesity is

defined as a BMI over 30. In 2020, President Trump weighed 243 pounds, and claimed to be 6'3" tall, nudging him into class I obesity, with a BMI just a hair over 30. Comedic actor John Candy had class II obesity, with a BMI of 39. Marlon Brando tipped the scales at 300 pounds when he showed up to play Colonel Kurtz in *Apocalypse Now*, to the dismay of director Francis Ford Coppola, who had wanted Kurtz to appear gaunt and haunted. Brando's BMI was over 43, well into the range of class III obesity.

BMI is unreliable in the extremely muscular. Arnold Schwarzenegger, in his steroidal heyday, had a BMI of 32, making him technically obese. BMI may also be misleading in the very short or very tall, or people with petite or husky frames. Some have suggested tweaking the BMI formula to correct for this, but these changes have not yet been widely adopted.

Which BMI is associated with the longest lifespan? In a meta-analysis of 230 studies by Dagfinn Aune and colleagues, all-cause mortality was lowest in people with BMIs from 23 to 27.5, or the high-normal to slightly overweight range. Obese and underweight BMIs were associated with higher risks of death, but surprisingly, so were BMIs in the low-normal range of 20-22.

One explanation is that these results were confounded by smokers and people with chronic disease in the low-normal BMI group. Because nicotine is an appetite suppressant, current and former smokers tend to be leaner than never-smokers, while having a higher risk of death. Patients with medical and psychiatric illness often have lower BMIs. People also may lose weight in the early stages of disease, before it becomes apparent that they are sick. It's not unusual for primary care doctors to see patients who are ecstatic that they've lost the weight that they've been trying to drop for years, only to diagnose them with cancer a few months later.

If you toss out smokers and people with chronic diseases, and just look at healthy never-smokers, the survival curve shifts down, with the longest life expectancy smack dab in the normal BMI range of 20 to 25. Unfortunately for the calorie restriction folks, underweight BMI is associated with a shorter lifespan. Compared to a BMI of 23, healthy never-smokers with a BMI of 17.5 had a 15% higher risk of dying. A Bowiesque BMI of 15 increases the risk of death by 48%.

Being overweight leads to modest decreases in survival. A BMI of 27.5 increases the risk of death by 11%, and a BMI of 30 is associated with a 24% higher chance of dying. Survival falls dramatically as BMIs climb into Santa Claus territory. A BMI of 35 is associated with a 66% increase in the risk of death, and a BMI of 40 increases your risk of dying by 137%.

As much as I would prefer to avoid it, it is impossible to discuss obesity and ideal body weight without tackling the messy subject of dietary fat. Until recently, fat, and especially saturated fat, was the leading villain in nutrition science. But dietary fat has been rehabilitated in recent years, and even saturated fat has undergone something of a heel-face turn.

Most saturated fat in the American diet comes from red meat and dairy products. Saturated fat is compact, and solid at room temperature; think lard, butter, and cooled bacon grease. Unlike saturated fats, unsaturated fats contain one double bond (monounsaturated fats) or several (polyunsaturated fats). Because of their double bonds, the molecules of unsaturated fats are kinked, and they don't stack nicely as saturated fats do. For this reason, unsaturated fats are liquid at room temperature. Canola, olive, and peanut oils mainly contain monounsaturated fats, while the fats in sunflower, sesame, soybean, and corn oils are largely polyunsaturated. Tropical plant oils, such as palm oil and coconut oil, are mostly saturated fat. There is more overlap than you might expect in the fat content of foods. For example, while pork and chicken contain saturated fat, they are also rich in oleic acid, the monounsaturated fat that is the major component of olive oil.

The scientist most responsible for the vilification of saturated fat was Ancel Keys, a physiologist at the University of Minnesota. (Keys' other claim to fame was the invention of the widely despised K-rations eaten by combat troops in World War II.) In the 1950s and 1960s, an era of near-universal cigarette smoking, heart attacks were alarmingly common. Saturated fat, which was known to hike up cholesterol, was a convenient scapegoat. Keys spearheaded a huge survey of diet, lifestyle, and coronary disease in the United States, Europe, and Japan, which became known as the Seven Countries Study. Not surprisingly, Keys found what he wanted to find: a link between saturated fat and heart attacks. This gave Keys powerful ammunition in his fight to cancel saturated fat.

But as Nina Teicholz points out in her book *The Big Fat Surprise*, the Seven Countries Study had troubling flaws. Data collection was patchy and incomplete, when it was not downright janky. For example, a big chunk of the Greek data that supposedly proved the superiority of a diet low in saturated fat was collected during Lent, when most of the subjects were fasting. And while saturated fat was indeed associated with higher rates of heart attacks, Keys failed to find a link between saturated fat and all-cause mortality.

The war on saturated fat had a disastrous unintended consequence: it drove consumers towards foods that seemed healthy, but were actually harmful. As butter and lard sales went down, consumption of margarine and shortening made from hydrogenated vegetable oils shot up. Unfortunately, industrial hydrogenation turns vegetable oils into trans fats, which are far deadlier than saturated fats. While saturated fats increase LDL, the bad cholesterol, they also give a modest boost to HDL, the good cholesterol. Trans fats have no redeeming qualities: they raise LDL, make HDL levels fall, fuel inflammation, and dampen blood vessel function, all of which increase the risk of stroke and heart attacks. (As of 2020, trans fats have largely been eliminated from the U.S. food chain.)

Keys' research gave all fats a bad reputation. Paradoxically, as fat-free foods soared in popularity, rates of obesity and type 2 diabetes skyrocketed. Fatty foods produce a pleasant feeling of satiety and fullness. On the other hand, fat-free products loaded with refined sugar and high-fructose corn syrup lead to wild swings in insulin and blood sugar levels. When you eat a meal rich in sugar, blood sugars rise, and provoke surges in insulin release. When blood sugars levels plunge in response, you feel hungry again. This vicious feedback loop leads to overeating, obesity, and burnout of the insulin-producing cells in the pancreas, with the development of type 2 diabetes.

The fearmongering over saturated fat seems to have been either grossly exaggerated, or at worst wholly mistaken. In recent meta-analyses, high saturated fat intakes were associated with either small increases or no changes in all-cause mortality. One large 2017 study, the PURE cohort, found that diets high in total fat and saturated fat were actually associated with lower all-cause mortality, while high carbohydrate intakes increased the risk of death. A recent Cochrane Collaboration meta-analysis found that clinical trials which tried to reduce saturated fat intake failed to lower all-cause mortality or cardiovascular mortality. While modest amounts of saturated fat in the diet are probably fine, monounsaturated fats and polyunsaturated fats from sources such as olive, canola, and corn oils are preferable, as they lead to significant drops in LDL cholesterol and are associated with lower rates of cardiovascular disease.

Dairy foods have been vilified for their high content of saturated fat, but they are also rich in calcium and potassium. In recent meta-analyses, milk, cheese, and yogurt appear to be neutral in their effects on all-cause mortality.

Omega-3 fatty acids are a special class of polyunsaturated fats, often referred to as fish oils. They are found in tree nuts as well as seafood, and play roles in brain function, cardiovascular health, and controlling inflammation. In the UK Biobank, a cohort study with over 400,000 participants, regular users of fish oil supplements had a 13% lower risk of death. However, this might be an example of healthy user bias. People who took fish oil supplements in this study were more active and tended to eat better, suggesting they were more health-conscious in general. Clinical trials of fish oil supplements have been disappointing, showing only mild benefit in preventing heart attacks, with no reduction in all-cause mortality. A recent meta-analysis found a modest reduction in all-cause mortality with regular fish consumption. This was more marked in Asia than in the United States and Europe, possibly due to the frequent consumption of less healthy deep-fried fish in Western nations.

What interventions are effective for weight loss? *Dieting* in the United States is a industry that takes in $72 billion annually, with scads of competing proprietary diets. These include the low-fat Ornish diet, the low-carbohydrate Atkins, South Beach, and Zone diets, and moderate macronutrient, or balanced diets, such Jenny Craig, Weight Watchers, and Nutrisystem. As these all seem to work equally well, finding a whole food diet that you like and can stick with is probably the most critical piece in a weight loss strategy. *Behavioral coaching* helps to lose weight in the short term, while *exercise* may be more important in the long run. (Compared to big brand-name programs, fitness and diet apps on smartphones are a cheaper way to create meal plans and track caloric intake and physical activity.)

The ketogenic or keto diet has soared in popularity of late. It is extremely high in fat, about 75%, with carbohydrates down to a bare minimum of 5%. (It was originally devised as a treatment for type 1 diabetes, before the discovery of insulin.) While it seems to be equivalent to other diet plans for weight loss, it has nuisance side effects that might reduce your chances of getting a prom date, such as halitosis, diarrhea, rashes, and muscle cramps. Another recent fad is the paleo diet, which purports to mimic the hearty folkways of our Stone Age ancestors. Paleo enthusiasts binge on red meat, and shun dairy, grains, and refined sugar. There are limited but favorable data from small clinical trials to support the use of paleo for weight loss.

Intermittent fasting has been suggested as a kinder, gentler way to get the metabolic benefits of calorie restriction, without the side effect of frailty. In 16:8 intermittent fasting, meals and snacks are compressed into eight hours, with the subject fasting for the other 16 hours of the day. A 12-week clinical trial in 116 overweight and obese participants found that the 16:8 group did not lose more weight than the group eating at regular meal times. Moreover, the 16:8 fasting group lost muscle mass and were more sluggish, as measured by an activity tracker. Glucose and cholesterol levels were similar in the two groups.

We've already seen how substituting *whole foods* for ultraprocessed foods promotes weight loss. In large American cohort studies, such as the Nurses' Health Study and the Health Professionals Follow-up Study, those who ate more fruits and nuts had healthier BMIs. Higher intake of vegetables was associated with weight loss, except for starchy vegetables with a high glycemic index, such as potatoes, peas, and corn, which were associated with weight gain. (As well, higher intakes of vegetables, fruits, and nuts are all associated with reduced all-cause mortality.)

A useful German word with no precise English equivalent is *kummerspeck*. Its literal translation is "grief bacon," weight gained from overeating due to sadness or stress. Measures that may help to *reduce emotional eating* include cognitive behavior therapy, mindfulness training, and treatment of underlying depression and anxiety.

Thanks to a sedentary lifestyle and a diet of ultraprocessed food with lavish amounts of high-fructose corn syrup, a staggering 43% of American adults are obese. However, there is one North American demographic with low obesity rates, despite meals high in saturated fat and refined sugar: the Amish. In one community of Old Order Amish farmers in Ontario, only 4% of adults were obese. Their secret appears to be nearly constant physical activity: men do over 18,000 steps per day, and women more than 14,000 steps per day (the U.S. average is 4,774 steps per day). If shoeing horses and tossing hay bales is not your thing, you can help control your weight by puttering around (the technical term for this is *nonexercise activity thermogenesis*). In the course of a day, you can burn calories by standing, walking, gardening, housecleaning, playing a musical instrument, knitting, fishing, woodworking, even plain old fidgeting.

It is conventional wisdom that breakfast is the most important meal of the day, and that a hearty meal to start the day helps you lose weight. Not surprisingly, this dogma has been embraced by makers of breakfast cereals. However, research shows that people who eat breakfast regularly tend to be heavier than people that *skip breakfast*. As well, starting to eat breakfast as a weight loss strategy may actually lead to weight gain.

Bariatric surgery, such as "stomach-stapling" and gastric bypass procedures, reduces the risk of death in the severely obese. In one meta-analysis, patients with class III obesity who had bariatric surgery had a 41% reduction in long-term all-cause mortality, compared to controls who did not undergo surgery.

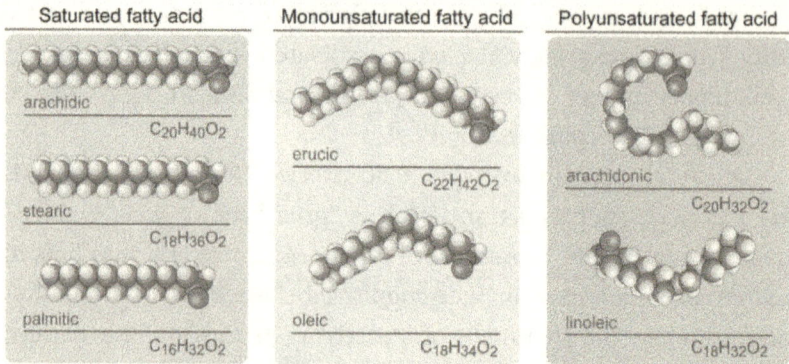

Saturated fatty acid	Monounsaturated fatty acid	Polyunsaturated fatty acid

arachidic $C_{20}H_{40}O_2$

erucic $C_{22}H_{42}O_2$

arachidonic $C_{20}H_{32}O_2$

stearic $C_{18}H_{36}O_2$

palmitic $C_{16}H_{32}O_2$

oleic $C_{18}H_{34}O_2$

linoleic $C_{18}H_{32}O_2$

Saturated fats have straight chains and stack easily, making them solid at room temperature, like lard and butter. Unsaturated fats have double bonds and are kinked, making them liquid at room temperature, like olive and canola oils. While unsaturated fats are probably healthier, saturated fats have been unfairly demonized for the past 60 years.

Lastly, there is some good news for the underweight and overweight: physical fitness may be a better predictor of lifespan than BMI. In a study of over 18,000 patients in the Veterans Affairs system who had exercise stress tests, highly fit patients in the underweight, normal weight, and overweight categories all had similar survival rates.

Body mass index classification

BMI	Nutritional status
Below 18.5	Underweight
18.5–24.9	Normal weight
25.0–29.9	Pre-obesity/overweight
30.0–34.9	Obesity class I
35.0–39.9	Obesity class II
Above 40	Obesity class III

CHAPTER 24

Moral Fiber

A high-fiber diet reduces the risk of obesity and metabolic syndrome.

In 1958, Dr. Ben Eiseman discovered the healing power of human feces. At the time, Eiseman was a surgeon at the Veterans Administration Hospital in Denver, treating septic patients with *Clostridioides difficile* colitis. In this infection, the normal, peaceable bacterial inhabitants of the large bowel are wiped out as collateral damage from antibiotics used to treat other infections. This allows the *C. difficile* bacterium to take over, transforming the colon into a leaky bag of toxins.

Eiseman, inspired by childhood memories of a sick animal eating its own stools, reasoned that feces from a healthy donor might repopulate the colon with good bacteria, and reverse the fatal effects of *C. difficile*. As Eiseman wrote 50 years later, "Those were days when if one had an idea, we simply tried it." One of Eiseman's residents was told to scavenge stools from women on the maternity wards. This pilfered poop was then given in enema form to four deathly ill patients with *C. difficile*. Their bloody diarrhea and abdominal pain resolved within 48 hours of the transpoosions, and all four made uneventful recoveries. Although Eiseman's work was forgotten for decades, fecal transplants are now known to be the most effective treatment for relapsing *C. difficile* colitis.

We contain as many bacteria in our guts as there are cells in our bodies. *C. difficile* colitis is an extreme example of a disease caused by disturbances in the bacterial populations, or microbiome, of the bowel. But Crohn's disease, allergic conditions, and even obesity may also be related to a microbiome that is out of whack. People with obesity tend to have gut microbiomes with low diversity, and a predominance of pro-inflammatory bacteria such as *Proteobacteria* and *Firmicutes*. (It is not yet clear whether these changes cause obesity, or whether they are just markers for an unhealthy diet of ultraprocessed food.)

The best way to maintain a healthy gut microbiome is a diet rich in fiber. Fiber, also known as roughage or bulk, is plant matter that humans are unable to digest. However, many types of fiber can be fermented and used for energy by gut bacteria. For this reason, fiber is sometimes called a prebiotic, as it promotes the growth of beneficial bacteria.

There are two kinds of fiber, soluble and insoluble. Insoluble fiber is a natural laxative. It prevents diverticular disease, in which an overworked colon weakens and develops bulging outpockets that bleed and get infected. Good sources of insoluble fiber include whole grains, bran, nuts, broccoli, cabbage, onions, green leafy vegetables, and fruit and vegetable skins.

Soluble fiber reacts with water in the intestines to form a gooey gelatinous material. This viscous goop slows down the absorption of glucose, avoiding harmful spikes in blood sugar after eating. Soluble fiber also lowers serum cholesterol. The liver converts some cholesterol to bile acids, which are secreted into the gut to help the body absorb fat. However, some bile acids get stuck in this soggy soluble fiber, and pass into the feces instead of being reabsorbed into the body. So the liver has to divert cholesterol into bile salt production, leading to lower levels of cholesterol in the blood. Soluble fiber is found in nuts, legumes such as peas and beans, oats, pectin-rich fruits such as apples, pears, apricots, peaches, and citrus, and vegetables such as Brussels sprouts, broccoli, and carrots.

High fiber intake is also associated with a lower risk of obesity. Fiber is filling and decreases appetite. It increases levels of hormones, such as cholecystokinin, that delay stomach emptying. Gut bacteria convert soluble fiber to short-chain fatty acids, which are absorbed into the blood and improve insulin sensitivity. This lowers levels of glucose and insulin, and reduces the risk of diabetes and metabolic syndrome.

In observational studies, dietary fiber is associated with reduced all-cause mortality. People in the top one-third of fiber intake have a 16% lower risk of death, compared to those in the bottom third. Each bump in daily fiber intake of 10 grams is associated with a 10% lower risk of death. (Ten grams is about the amount of fiber you'd get from a bowl of bran cereal, a generous serving of beans, or two large apples with the skin on.)

CHAPTER 25

Only the Good Die Old

Conscientious people live longer.

In 1921, Lewis Terman, a Stanford psychologist, began a study of 1500 California school children with IQs in the genius range. Terman followed these prodigies for decades, collecting huge amounts of information. Among other things, his overstuffed files included personality ratings of the students, completed by their parents and teachers.

The Terman Study of the Gifted puttered along for the next 80 years, continuing after Terman's death. Several so-called "Termites" became famous, such as anti-cholesterol zealot Ancel Keys, Jess Oppenheimer, the showrunner for *I Love Lucy*, and Edward Dmytryk, who directed Humphrey Bogart in *The Caine Mutiny*. Some went into law, finance, engineering, and academia, while others became clerks, cops, and truck drivers.

In 1990, two psychologists, Howard Friedman and Leslie Martin, realized that the Terman Study might be a motherlode of data about personality and health. Conventional wisdom at that time held that laid-back people lived longer, while those who toiled away died young. In fact, Friedman and Martin found exactly the opposite. Kids who were conscientious—that is, scrupulous, driven, and hardworking—usually grew up to be adults with prosperous careers, happy marriages, and long lifespans. On the other hand, carefree, happy-go-lucky students were liable to underachieve at work, flounder in their marriages, and die young.

Friedman and Martin's findings have been validated in several other studies. A meta-analysis of 19 cohorts with nearly 9,000 participants found a consistent association of conscientiousness with lower all-cause mortality. Two studies not included in this meta-analysis had similar results. In the Baltimore Longitudinal Study of Aging, a cohort of nearly 2,400 people followed for five decades, conscientiousness was the personality attribute most tightly correlated with longevity. The Harvard Grant Study enrolled 268 Harvard sophomores between 1938 and 1942, and subjected them to an intensive battery of tests and interviews. (No female students were enrolled, because at that time Harvard didn't have any.) Even amongst this privileged group, being conscientious was a strong predictor of lifespan. Harvard men who scored strongly in perseverance and self-motivation lived ten years longer on average than those who did not. In fact, conscientiousness was a better predictor of longevity than parental wealth, exercise, obesity, or happiness in childhood.

The popular press often touts studies claiming that the secret of long life is to just be happy, as if blissfulness was a switch that could be turned on and off. In reality, the relationship between happiness and longevity is murky. Neither the Terman Study of the Gifted nor the Harvard Grant Study found that a happy childhood was associated with longer lifespan. In fact, the Terman Study found exactly the opposite: the happiest kids tended to have the shortest lives, probably because they were the least conscientious. Data is mixed on the health value of happiness in later life. In the English Longitudinal Study of Aging, happiness was associated with longer life expectancy, while in the UK Million Women Study, it was not.

Furthermore, happiness is not static through the life course. For the average American, happiness typically has a first peak, around the age of 20. It then declines slowly, bottoming out in middle age, when many people feel overworked and underpaid, and are stressed out by teenage kids and ailing parents. From this nadir, happiness rises again, reaching a second peak in old age. By age 65, the average person is happier than they were at age 20, despite being less healthy. (At least, this is the pattern in well-off English-speaking countries. In Eastern Europe and the former Soviet Union, there is a long continuous decline in happiness over the life course, from age 20 onward.)

Why might conscientiousness be more important than happiness for longevity? For one thing, disciplined and hardworking people put themselves in a better position to live longer. They tend to have greater educational attainment, higher socioeconomic status, and stronger relationships, all of which are associated with longevity. Secondly, they have better coping and problem-solving skills, leading to less physiological stress and hormonal wear-and-tear. Finally, they have healthier behaviors. By and large, they eat better, exercise more, heed medical advice, and don't smoke or booze up.

Friedman and Martin found that conscientiousness could change during the life course. Serious and sober children could become feckless and unreliable grownups, while wild kids might mature into steady and dependable adults. The Termites who showed discipline for only part of their life history lived longer, on average, than those who were never conscientious, but not as long as those with lifelong self-control.

How can one become more conscientious? There is moderate evidence for techniques that teach patients to behave and think like conscientious people do. In *cognitive-behavioral therapy*, subjects work with a therapist to learn how to avoid self-defeating behaviors and reinforce successful ones. *Meta-cognitive techniques* focus on goals, how to reach them, and how to draw up contingency plans if the first one doesn't work out. In *cognitive remediation*, which was originally developed for survivors of traumatic brain injury, subjects do brain exercises to improve memory, attention, and executive function.

You may ask yourself: health benefits aside, why bother with being conscientious? Is it worth the effort and the sacrifice? Why not just live for today? Without getting into questions of wherein lies the Good and the Right, which are beyond the scope of this book, the simplest answer is that people who are conscientious are more likely to flourish over the long run. Data from both the Terman Study from the Gifted and the Harvard Grant Study suggest that happiness is a byproduct of responsible living. Conscientious people make choices that lead to strong relationships, rewarding careers, and better well-being. In life's marathon, the conscientious are generally healthier, and happier too.

CHAPTER 26

Marriage Story

Stable marriages and partnerships prolong lifespan. This is true for both sexes, but especially so for men.

Marriage is the best state for a man in general.

—Samuel Johnson

No matter how a man alone ain't got no bloody fucking chance.

—Hemingway, *To Have and Have Not*

From the point of view of mortality, marriage is of much less benefit to women than to men, though for the sake of long life it is sufficient to be well worth considering.

—*JAMA*, "Comparative Mortality of Married and Single Persons," July 19, 1913

And if you couldn't be loved, the next best thing was to be let alone.

—Lucy Maud Montgomery, *Jane of Lantern Hill*

One of my most valuable learning experiences as a trainee in internal medicine was making house calls. Unless you see patients where they live, you may be clueless as to how they are really doing, and what pitfalls they face on their road to health.

One day, my preceptor asked me to check on a gentleman I'll call Frank X, whose recent clinic attendance had been erratic. Frank had toiled for years, Bartleby-like, in a low-level clerical job. A divorce in middle age left him bitter, broke, and estranged from friends and family. Left to his own devices, he took early retirement, and went alarmingly to seed.

Frank lived in an apartment building of faded brick in the outer reaches of Boston. I stood in the shabby vestibule and pressed the tinny buzzer, with no response. I turned to leave, when I realized that I might contrive to see into Frank's front window from the edge of the stoop. In a typically dubious decision, I hung off the outside of the railing with one hand, while balancing on the verge of the platform. Leaning to the side, I saw Frank in an undershirt, motionless in a dilapidated armchair. *Oh God, he's dead*, I thought. With my free hand I pounded frantically on the window. Frank, blessedly, began to stir, trying and failing to get to his feet, repeatedly foiled by gravity.

At length, Frank made it upright long enough to beep me in, and staggered back to his armchair. A sorry midden of takeout containers and crushed Coors cans sprawled across the battered oak floors. The air stank of stale beer, with fragrance notes of sweat and urine. Although Frank was clearly intoxicated, he was able to respond to my suggestion to go to the hospital with a colorful enjoinder to perform the anatomically impossible. Having ascertained that Frank's pulse and blood pressure were adequate to sustain life, I left in a state of professional befuddlement. (We eventually succeeded in getting Frank into a residential detox.)

A considerable body of evidence shows that married people are healthier and live longer than singles. In a 2020 meta-analysis of 21 studies involving nearly 8 million people, all-cause mortality was 22% higher in unmarried women, and a whopping 46% higher in unmarried men. (As all married women know, men benefit more from marriage than women do.) Heart attack, stroke, and cancer are all more common in singles than in married people. A Danish study also suggests that cohabitation with a member of the opposite sex, or what was known in my Baptist hometown as "living in sin" or "shacking up," has similar health benefits to marriage. Why might the divorced, separated, and never married have a higher risk of death, compared to people in long-term relationships?

There are two major explanations for the longer lifespans of married people. The first is that marriage has biological benefits that delay aging and prolong life. The second theory is that traits and behaviors that lead to good marriages also favor long life spans. Happily married folks differ in temperament and behavior from those who get divorced, or never marry at all. Conversely, the Frank Xs of the world may have unhealthy lifestyles and personalities that put them at risk for failed relationships *and* shorter lives. There is probably truth to both these theories.

In cohort studies, unmarried men and women are more likely to have low socioeconomic status, and are more prone to have poor health behaviors, such as smoking. Single men, but not single women, tend to be less educated. Studies try to adjust for these factors, but there may be residual confounding that makes marriage look better for you than it actually is.

The personal qualities that keep a marriage humming along may also help people to live longer. Support for this comes from the eight decades of data on the Termites, the high-IQ kids from Lewis Terman's Study of the Gifted. Termites who were driven and conscientious were more likely to live long, and succeed in both work and love. On the other hand, carefree Termites tended to have mediocre careers, failed marriages, and early deaths.

The Termites who got divorced had a higher risk of death than those who stayed married. But in this unusual population of highly intelligent men and women, those who never married lived as long as the stably married people, provided they had robust social networks. This suggests that an abundance of other social ties can provide a similar degree of support as marriage.

While some of the mortality penalty for singles may be the result of personality problems and self-sabotage, marriage probably does reduce your risk of dying. Spousal encouragement, or perhaps nagging, seems to promote healthy behaviors. Compared to singles, couples are more likely to eat whole foods and heed medical advice. A more critical benefit is social support. Married people can draw on shared social networks in times of need, while the love of a spouse buffers against anguish and despair, which are alarmingly common in singles. In a Japanese study, 22% of the never married felt hopeless, while 41% of divorced men and 52% of divorced women felt unfulfilled. Psychological distress is associated with our old foes, the stress hormones cortisol, epinephrine, and norepinephrine, which may lead to hypertension, cardiovascular disease, and diabetes.

It makes sense that happy marriages prolong life, but what about miserable ones? We men are so feckless and so inept at taking care of ourselves that even a bad marriage is better for us than no marriage at all. According to a study by Heejeong Choi and Nadine Marks at Penn State, men in high-conflict marriages still live longer than single men. This is especially true for men with low incomes. Matters are different for women, who tend to have healthier lifestyles and sturdier social networks. There is zero survival benefit for a low-income woman in a high-conflict marriage. In fact, she may be less stressed and live longer if she gets a divorce. Conversely, women in high-conflict marriages in high-income households seem to live a little longer overall than single women with high incomes. Apparently, the soothing effects of affluence can paper over the flaws of a defective marriage.

Although widows and widowers have a higher risk of death than married people, they are better off than the divorced, separated, or never married. Compared to married men, the risk of all-cause mortality is 67% higher in never-married men, 59% higher in divorced or separated men, but only 30% higher in widowers. Findings in women are similar, but the absolute benefit of marriage is lower. All-cause mortality is 46% higher in never-married women, 27% higher in divorced or separated women, and only 14% higher in widows, compared to married women. Because of the stress of grief, the risk of death is high in the first six months after losing a spouse, but it fades away thereafter. Presumably, widows and widowers do better over the longer term than the divorced or never married because their social networks and finances are less disrupted.

Loneliness and divorce seem to accelerate aging. In a cohort of over 10,000 Swedes, those who lived alone had, on average, significantly shorter telomeres than those who were married or living together. Another study suggested that marital disruption may be worse than solitude in speeding aging. In an American cohort of over 3,500 people, those who were divorced, separated, and widowed had shorter telomeres than the never married and the continuously married. These findings were still significant after adjusting for personality factors, BMI, smoking, and childhood and lifetime traumatic events. In this study, the scars that divorce left at a cellular level seemed to be permanent. Telomere shortening was similar among the divorced and remarried, compared to the divorced and still single. This is consistent with other data showing that divorce does lasting damage to life span, and that multiple divorces seem to have additive effects in reducing life expectancy.

Same-sex marriage, like opposite-sex marriage, seems to be associated with better health. In the United States, where many people are covered by their spouse's health insurance plan, this may be partly due to improved access to medical care. Support from partners and shared social networks likely also play a role. LGBT persons in California who were married or in domestic partnerships have less psychological distress than LGBT singles. In the year after same-sex marriage was legally recognized in Massachusetts, sexual minorities required significantly fewer medical and mental health clinic visits. (These benefits were similar in married and single LGBT patients, suggesting that a sense of empowerment and reduced stigma was also important.)

CHAPTER 27

Gotta Serve Somebody

Have a reason to get out of bed in the morning.

If you have your why for life, then you can get along with
almost any how.

—Friedrich Nietzsche, *Twilight of the Idols*

Viktor Frankl was a world expert on suicide. Oddly enough, this may
have helped him to survive the Holocaust. Before the war, Frankl
was a psychiatrist with a focus on the treatment of the suicidal. His
interest was not the product of chance. As a young man, he had often
been overwhelmed by depression. He later claimed this made him
immune to nihilism.

From 1933 until 1937, Frankl oversaw the female suicide ward
at the Steinhof Psychiatric Hospital in Vienna. As a Jew, Frankl was
fired after the Nazi takeover, but he eventually became the head of
neurology at the Rothschild, Vienna's Jewish hospital. As many as
1,200 Viennese Jews committed suicide during the Nazi era. Frankl
made heroic if misbegotten efforts to revive patients that had over-
dosed on sleeping pills, going so far as to inject amphetamines directly into the fluid cavities of the brain.

In September 1942, Frankl and his family were deported to the
Theresienstadt ghetto, in what is now the Czech Republic. While

there, he ran what we would now call a suicide crisis service, and counselled traumatized new arrivals to the ghetto. He was sent to Auschwitz in October 1944, and finally transferred to a subcamp of Dachau, from which he was liberated at the end of World War II. Most of his immediate family perished in the Holocaust, including his wife, brother, and both parents.

The inmates of Dachau were beaten and brutalized, starved, worked to the point of collapse, and kept in filthy conditions that spread dysentery and typhus. According to Frankl, men sometimes succumbed to despair. This was much feared, and inevitably fatal: "The prisoner who had lost faith in the future—his future—was doomed." This crisis usually came on suddenly, with the man refusing to leave his hard wooden bunk in the morning to report to the parade grounds. Threats, pleas, and blows were equally futile. The prisoner would even turn down attempts to take him to sickbay for respite care.

In Dachau, Frankl was asked to speak to would-be suicides, or men who had lost hope. His approach to this difficult task was to focus on their reasons for living. He asked them to imagine a future after the war, when they might reunite with their families and pursue creative work. He urged them to recall their peak moments in life, all their joys and longings and exaltations. Finally, he encouraged them to find meaning by acting with decency and courage in the face of senseless suffering and cruelty. After the war, this approach became the basis of Frankl's logotherapy, which held that the quest for purpose in life, rather than the pursuit of pleasure, was the most important and uniquely human drive.

If searching for reasons to live makes us human, finding them may lead to longer life. In Japan, purpose in life is known as *ikigai*, a term that also means delight in being alive. If one's *ikigai* is work, it is work that is done gladly. For older generations, *ikigai* typically involves service to family and community; for the young, it more often entails self-realization and mastery. In one Japanese cohort study, subjects with no *ikigai* had a 50% higher risk of dying. Other studies in Japan and the United States have had similar findings. A meta-analysis of ten studies with over 136,000 subjects found that having purpose in life was associated with a 17% lower risk of death, even after adjusting for confounding factors such as exercise, smoking, and underlying medical conditions. The biological mechanisms responsible are unknown, but might involve the usual suspects of lower levels of stress hormones and inflammation, as well as residual confounding from better health behaviors.

Reasons to live may be quite specific in the old and ill. Sick patients may be determined to survive until some special occasion, such as a 90th birthday, or the wedding of a favorite grandchild. There is a belief that those holding onto life to reach some milestone are at high risk of dying soon thereafter, like a marathoner collapsing at the finish line. The evidence for this catch-up mortality is not robust. In fact, a large Swiss study showed that people were 14% more likely to die *on* their birthday, with the risk of death being normal in the week after a birthday. Deaths from strokes, heart attacks, and suicide are more common on birthdays. One possible explanation is mortality salience, or the birthday blues: the unwelcome intrusion into consciousness of the inevitability of death. Fatal falls and accidents are also more frequent on birthdays, suggesting a supporting role for alcohol. (Frankl reported catch-up mortality in Dachau. Many prisoners had clung to life in the forlorn hope that the war would end by Christmas Day, 1944. In the following week, when it became clear that this was not the case, the death rate in the camp soared.)

Religion, purpose, and longevity seem to be intertwined. A large and consistent body of evidence suggests that regular churchgoers have a lower risk of death than the ungodly. In an older meta-analysis of 42 studies with nearly 126,000 participants, the risk of death was 22% higher in people who were not religious, compared to the devout. A more recent prospective study with nearly 90,000 participants in three different cohorts had similar findings. After adjusting for baseline demographics and health status, those who attended religious services at least weekly had a 26% lower risk of death, compared to never-attenders. The most likely explanation is that churchgoers have healthier behaviors, as well as better social adjustment. Those who went to religious services religiously were 34% less likely to be heavy drinkers, and 29% less likely to smoke. They also had larger social networks, a stronger sense of purpose in life, and greater life satisfaction. Anxiety, hopelessness, and loneliness were less common in churchgoers. They were also less likely to be depressed, a protective effect that was especially robust in young adults.

For those who aren't into hymnals and holy water, are there secular alternatives with similar benefits? Volunteering can be particularly valuable for retirees, who may find renewed life purpose as their roles as parents and breadwinners begin to fade. Where health is concerned, it may truly be better to give than to receive. In one meta-analysis, older adults who did volunteer work had a 24% lower risk of death. This study controlled for several variables, including baseline health status, which helped to rule out reverse causation (that is, the possibility that volunteers lived longer because they were healthier than non-volunteers, who may have been too sick to take on added work). Volunteering creates opportunities for social contact, physical activity, and brain stimulation, and is associated with lower risks of depression, disability, and dementia. The health benefits of volunteering seem to max out at a threshold of 100 hours per year.

Mammals are hardwired to be caregivers, especially long-lived mammals like humans, so it may not be surprising that altruism and unselfish behavior seem to buffer stress (that is, as long as the caregiver is not overwhelmed and burnt out, as happens with spouses of demented or terminally ill patients). Blood pressure seems to be especially responsive to prosocial behavior. In one study, volunteers were randomized to either write a letter of support to a friend in trouble, or a description of the route they took to get to work or school. They were then put through a stressful simulated job interview, in which they had to pitch themselves to a panel of judges. The subjects who wrote letters of support had lower blood pressures during the hiring scenario, and their blood pressures came back to normal more quickly after the interview was over. In another study, people who gave generously to charity had lower blood pressures than cheapskates and skinflints when seen in follow-up two years later (the data were adjusted for socioeconomic status and other variables).

The stress-relieving effect of altruistic behavior actually can be seen on brain imaging, using a functional MRI scanner. When volunteers performed tasks that gave them a chance to win money for friends, fMRI scans showed lower activity in parts of the brain that perceive threats and increase stress, such as the amygdala, and higher activity in the brain's reward or feel-good centers, such as the ventral striatum.

CHAPTER 28

Java Jive

Moderate amounts of coffee and tea are safe and may prolong life.

A Potion stimulating rebellion and immoderate desires.

— Thomas Pynchon, *Mason & Dixon*

One of the few things that still unites Americans is the love of a cup of joe. Seventy-five percent of American adults drink coffee at least occasionally, and 49% drink it daily. Rates of coffee drinking are similar in men and women, in college graduates and high school dropouts, and in those with high and low household incomes. While coffee is popular across the board in the U.S., there are demographic differences in intake. People drink more as they get older, with consumption maxing out between 50 and 60 years of age. As well, 80% of Latino Americans and 76% of white Americans drink coffee, compared to only 61% of black Americans. White folks *really* like their jamocha. Their average daily coffee consumption is double that of black and Latino Americans.

The American love affair with coffee began with the Boston Tea Party, when the rebels gave up tea to dodge British taxes. Although fancy brews are now a fetish of the bourgeoisie, java and revolt were intertwined for centuries. The French Revolution began in a hipster coffee shop on July 12, 1789, when Camille Desmoulins jumped on top of a table at the Café Foy in Paris. Desmoulins was 26 years old, a struggling journalist whose law career had failed because of his severe stammer. Now, hopped up on caffeine and adrenaline, his stutter vanished, and he spoke to the crowd in a torrent of eloquence. The mob rushed off to get muskets and swords, and the Bastille was stormed two days later.

Conservatives reacted with alarm when coffee and tea exploded in popularity in Europe in the 17th century. Charles II thought that the coffeehouses of England were nurseries of rebellion, and tried to shut them down in 1675. Others saw the dark brews as the workings of a sinister conspiracy. German physician Simon Pauli claimed that the traffic in coffee and tea was an Asiatic plot to sap European men of their precious bodily fluids, leaving them in a state of "effeminacy and impotence."

The new beverages also had staunch defenders. In 1678, Dr. Cornelius Bontekoe told his patients that industrial quantities of tea were completely safe, and would rid them of headaches and kidney stones. His choice of words was not entirely reassuring. "I have no scruple in advising people to drink fifty or a hundred or two hundred cups at a time. I have often drunk as many in a morning or an afternoon, and many people with me, of whom not a single one has died yet." Bontekoe's credibility took a hit when critics revealed that he was on the take from Big Tea. The good doctor was getting kickbacks from the Dutch East India Company, a huge tea importer, and the world's largest corporation at the time.

Concerns that coffee caused cancer and cardiovascular disease lingered well into the twentieth century. For the most part, these worries aren't worth a hill of coffee beans. They arose for two reasons. First, people who drink coffee are more likely to smoke. Until smoking rates dropped in recent decades, it was difficult to disentangle the effects of coffee from those of cigarettes. The other issue is that unfiltered coffee contains small amounts of a fat called cafestol. This chemical raises cholesterol levels by about 10%. Standard paper filters remove almost all the cafestol from coffee. However, unfiltered coffees do contain cafestol, and could increase your risk of heart disease. These include Greek and Turkish coffee, which is boiled with finely ground beans, and coffee made with a cafetière, or French press. (There is also cafestol in espresso, but this is unlikely to mess with your cholesterol, unless you are drinking several shots per day.)

Moderate consumption of coffee seems to come with several health perks. In a recent review, daily consumption of three to four cups of coffee per day was associated with a 17% reduction in all-cause mortality, a 16% reduction in the risk of death from heart attacks, and a 30% reduction in death from stroke. It was also associated with lower risks of type 2 diabetes, liver disease, Alzheimer's dementia, Parkinson's disease, and cancer. Possible harms include higher rates of miscarriage, low birth weight, and osteoporotic fractures in women.

If the health benefits of coffee are real, and not merely confounding from coffee bingeing by white people of high socioeconomic status, caffeine might be the reason why. Caffeine prevents a molecule called cyclic AMP from being broken down. When a lot of cyclic AMP is floating around in a cell, it increases the cell's basal metabolic rate, or the amount of energy the cell uses at rest. A cell pumped up on caffeine is like a car engine with a high idle, burning extra gas without moving. Caffeine also lowers blood glucose, burns off fat, decreases appetite, and increases energy expenditure during exercise.

Laboratory studies have examined the impact of a 300 mg dose of caffeine on metabolism. (That's the amount of caffeine in one 16-ounce Starbucks grande, two 14-ounce Tim Hortons medium coffees, or six cups of black tea.) In young men, this much caffeine boosts basal metabolic rate by 10-15% for at least two hours. This translates to about 20 wasted calories per day. That might not seem like a big deal. However, if those 20 calories were converted to fat instead, you'd gain two pounds in a year, and 20 pounds over a decade. This may be one reason why coffee is associated with lower risks of obesity and type 2 diabetes.

High intake of decaffeinated coffee has also been associated with lower all-cause mortality. This could be due to the many antioxidants found in both regular and decaf coffee, such as chlorogenic acid, which may lower blood pressure and improve blood glucose levels. It is also possible that the apparent benefit of decaf may be something of an illusion. Most people who drink decaf also drink a fair amount of caffeinated coffee, and many studies don't adjust very well for this. It's also been shown, in a 2017 study by Tetsuro Tsujimoto and colleagues, that people who drink more decaf coffee tend to take in more caffeine. This is partly because decaffeinated coffee is not caffeine-free. A cup of decaf contains as much as 15 mg of caffeine. People who drink decaf may also get caffeine from other sources, such as tea, soda, energy drinks, and chocolate.

Tea, which is similar to coffee in its content of caffeine and antioxidants, has also been associated with improved survival. In one meta-analysis, with most data coming from Asia and Europe, each daily cup of tea was associated with a 2% lower risk of death. Black tea and green tea seem to be equally beneficial.

I should not have to point this out, but just to be absolutely clear, the potential health benefits of coffee and tea are associated with *oral* consumption. Coffee should not be inserted into other bodily orifices. Don't wind up like the woman from Detroit who performed a coffee enema on herself at the behest of her naturopathic physician, and wound up with a massive case of proctocolitis.

CHAPTER 29

Brain Drain

*Stave off dementia by staying physically, socially,
and intellectually active.*

On November 25, 1901, a railwayman brought his wife to the Frankfurt Asylum for the Insane, a dismal Gothic heap better known by its nickname of Castle Bedlam. The woman, who was 51 years old and whose name was Auguste Deter, would die in this grim place four years later. In photos from the asylum, she is a haggard woman in a coarsely woven nightgown, with the look of troubled bafflement characteristic of dementia. Although she came from a poor family, Auguste was an educated woman. She had been an ordinary, dutiful housewife until a few months before, when her mind grew cloudy. At first, she got lost in familiar neighborhoods, and struggled with everyday tasks, such as cooking and cleaning. Then her behavior took a turn for the bizarre. She became paranoid, hid things, dragged the washing through the streets. She fought with neighbors and accused her husband of infidelity. At nightfall she screamed that assassins were coming to kill her.

When Auguste came to Castle Bedlam, she was examined by Alois Alzheimer, a heavy-set Bavarian whose playful manner belied the sinister dueling scars on his face. Alzheimer, whose major contribution to medical science until that point had been a doctoral thesis on the manufacture of earwax, was most struck by Auguste's near-total loss of short-term memory. She named objects that were shown to her, but forgot them as soon as they were taken from her sight. She was still able to read and write, but could only take dictation one word at a time, being unable to retain an entire sentence.

Alzheimer moved on to a more prestigious post, but he kept tabs on the unfortunate Frau Deter. When she succumbed to bedsores and pneumonia, like many a dementia patient before and since, Alzheimer arranged for her pickled brain to be shipped to his laboratory in Munich. He stained thin slices of her cerebral cortex with silver solution to bring out the delicate tracery of neurons and synapses. Under the microscope, her brain was studded with blobs of protein. A third of the neurons had died, and the survivors were choked with clumps of fibers that looked like snarled fishing lines. These findings, amyloid plaques and neurofibrillary tangles, are typical of what we now call Alzheimer's disease, the most common form of dementia.

What caused the lesions in Frau Deter's brain? At heart, Alzheimer's disease is a hoarding problem. Amyloid plaques and neurofibrillary tangles are toxic clutter, a buildup of misshapen proteins that the brain is unable to get rid of. Plaques arise from an abnormal version of a protein called amyloid-beta, and tangles from a misfolded form of the tau protein. (The correlation between plaque size and dementia severity is not strong. In fact, small bits of amyloid-beta may cause more damage than big plaques.) Inflammation, oxidative stress, and narrowed blood vessels also have roles in the development of Alzheimer's disease. When Alzheimer's develops at younger ages, as in Auguste Deter, genetic factors are often in play.

Alzheimer's disease is sometimes erroneously called old-timer's disease. (This is an excellent example of an eggcorn, a word misheard as a plausible substitute.) Not surprisingly, the relationship between Alzheimer's disease and advanced age is strong. Old cells are poor at tidying up free radicals and malformed proteins. The risk of Alzheimer's disease doubles every five years after age 65. New diagnoses of Alzheimer's disease level off after age 95, although the chance of getting dementia from other causes, such as mini-strokes, continues to climb in the super-aged. However, the risk for dementia is not set in stone. In fact, rates of dementia at any given age seems to have fallen in recent decades, perhaps related to more education, tighter control of high blood pressure, and decreased smoking.

What might delay the onset of dementia? *Educational achievement* seems to reduce the risk of dementia and all-cause mortality, although this is difficult to tease out from the protective effects of affluence, healthier lifestyles, and access to medical care that typically go with it. In one study, educational attainment was a better predictor of telomere length than socioeconomic status. This could be because low educational achievement is often a marker for a stressful childhood, which is associated with premature aging. Conversely, higher educational levels are associated with better problem-solving skills, which reduce biological stress and aging.

While educational attainment may postpone Alzheimer's disease, there is evidence that dementia is more aggressive in the highly educated once it is diagnosed. This is probably because people with greater cognitive reserve conceal or compensate for the effects of dementia until the disease is farther advanced.

Those who are not inclined to pursue a Ph.D. in String Theory can try *stimulating leisure activities.* In a 2003 study, the activities associated with the greatest reductions in dementia risk in adults over the age of 75 were reading, playing board games, playing a musical instrument, and dancing. Crossword puzzlers in the Bronx Aging Study had a delay in memory decline of 2.5 years, compared to elderly patients who did not do crossword puzzles. In the Monongahela Valley Independent Elders Survey (MoVIES) study, a high time commitment to reading and other hobbies protected against dementia in the elderly. Computerized brain training has been touted as a way to prevent cognitive decline, but the evidence for this is currently inconclusive.

Building brainpower throughout the lifespan may be the most effective strategy to avoid dementia. In a longitudinal cohort of 498 adults born in 1936 who took the Scottish Mental Survey in 1947, the lowest dementia risk was seen in those with a pattern of lifelong mental activity, as measured by engagement in reading, problem solving, abstract thought, and intellectual curiosity. This is consistent with other data that successful aging starts early, by avoiding physical and mental middle-aged dry rot. It is not realistic, after a lifetime of intellectual laziness, to expect that picking up a saxophone or a book of sudoku puzzles at age 75 will ward off dementia.

The brain is thirstier for blood than a vampire in the Sahara. It guzzles glucose and oxygen, and sucks up about 20% of cardiac output. As you'd expect, it is vulnerable to injury from inadequate blood flow. High blood pressure increases the risk for all types of dementia. However, it has a particular link to vascular dementia, in which the white matter, the wiring that connects different parts of the brain, is frayed and broken. The arterioles that feed the white matter are long and thin, and prone to damage from longstanding hypertension. In the SPRINT-MIND trial, it was shown that *tight blood pressure control*, with a target systolic blood pressure of less than 120 mm Hg, reduced the risk of developing either dementia or mild cognitive impairment, compared to a systolic blood pressure target of less than 140 mm Hg. (However, fainting episodes were more common in patients with lower blood pressure targets.)

Aerobic exercise seems to slow brain aging. In observational studies, regular vigorous physical activity (hard enough to break a sweat) is associated with lower risks of dementia. Exercise decreases inflammation and increases blood flow to the cerebral cortex. It also leads to surges in the production of brain-derived neurotrophic factor (BDNF). This protein, hyped by psychiatrist John Ratey as "Miracle-Gro for the brain," promotes the repair and survival of nerve cells. It even makes new neurons sprout up in the hippocampus, the brain's memory center, something that was once thought to be impossible.

In one clinical trial of the effects of aerobic exercise on the brain, 120 older adults were randomized to either moderate-intensity aerobic exercise (40-minute sessions, three days a week), or a control group that did stretching exercises. At the end of one year, the aerobic exercise group had a 2% increase in the volume of the hippocampus, as measured by magnetic resonance imaging (MRI). Those who did only stretching exercises had a 1.4% decrease in hippocampal size. (This is the usual yearly shrinkage of the hippocampus in older adults.)

Several studies have shown that *social contact* is associated with a lower risk of dementia. For example, in a prospective study of nearly 14,000 older Japanese adults followed for nine years, those who were highly socially connected were nearly 46% less likely to develop dementia than those who were most isolated. (This is a good example of a study that might be prone to reverse causation. That is, some people might be solitary because they already have early dementia, making it harder for them to keep up their social networks. The authors adjusted for this by running an analysis that excluded people who were diagnosed with dementia within three years of the beginning of the study. This had minimal effects on the results.)

If you've been to a few too many Sonic Youth or Motörhead concerts, you might need *hearing aids.* Prospective studies have shown that hearing loss increases dementia risk, presumably by worsening social isolation. Use of properly functioning hearing aids in the hearing impaired seems to decrease dementia risk.

There are also things you should avoid to reduce your chance of dementia. *Sleep disturbances*, both too much and too little sleep, are associated with dementia. The brain has a recently discovered waste disposal system, known as the glymphatics, that is most active in deep sleep. Not enough deep sleep may lead to buildup of amyloid-beta and other toxic proteins. What about the association between excess sleep duration and dementia? People with sleep apnea may sleep for long periods. However, their sleep is fragmented and low-quality, without the stages of deep sleep that seem to be crucial for brain repair.

Traumatic brain injury increases the risk of dementia, so try to avoid a bonk on the noggin. *Cigarette smoking* increases your risk of most bad things, including dementia. Even if you're older, quitting smoking reduces dementia risk. *Heavy alcohol use* leads to dementia by damaging the hippocampus. *Obesity*, defined as BMI > 30, increases dementia risk (however, merely being overweight does not). Weight loss in the obese improves attention and memory. *Diabetes* predisposes to dementia, with the risk increasing with diabetes severity and duration. Finally, *air pollution* may lead to dementia by damaging blood vessels and kindling inflammation in the brain. Perhaps poor Frau Deter breathed in too much soot from a coal-burning stove in a stuffy kitchen.

CHAPTER 30

Running Up That Hill

Do 150 minutes of moderate aerobic activity, or 75 minutes of vigorous aerobic activity, every week.

The oldest person who ever lived, Jeanne Calment, died in August 1997 in Arles, the French city where she had been born 122 years earlier. By the time of her death, Jeanne had become a national symbol of resilience and *joie de vivre*. Calment made good copy for reporters, who ate up her stories and one-liners. When she was 119, an interviewer asked, "Maybe I'll see you next year?" She answered, "Why not? You don't seem to be in such bad health." She told of meeting Vincent van Gogh when he was buying canvas in her future husband's dry goods shop. (She was unimpressed with the artist, whom she remembered as a rude and tetchy drunk.) At the age of 94, she signed a contract with a notary public named André-François Raffray, giving him ownership of her apartment at her death, as long as he paid her 2,500 francs a month while she was alive. This proved to be a spectacularly poor investment for Raffray. When the notary complained of her extraordinary longevity, she replied, "Excuse me if I'm clinging on to life, but my parents wove me from tight thread." When Raffray expired at the tender age of 77, his widow was on the hook for the payments for another two years, until Calment finally passed on.

The press liked to play up Calment's rebellious side, portraying her as a salty old broad with a sharp tongue who liked her chocolate, and sneaked the occasional Gauloise or glass of port. In truth, while

Calment had an independent streak, she came from a bourgeois and conventional background, with many traits conducive to long life. Her socioeconomic status was high. Her father was a prosperous shipbuilder, and her husband a successful merchant. She had household servants for much of her life, and never felt poverty's pinch. She was a regular churchgoer who prayed every day at St. Trophime's Cathedral. She was female and short, with an adult height of 4' 11" (150 cm), and a BMI of 20. Her family history of longevity was robust. She followed a typical Mediterranean diet, rich in fruit, olive oil, and garlic (she had a special fondness for aioli). She was cultured, and engaged in several activities to stimulate her mind, such as painting, playing the piano, reading, crosswords, and attending the opera in Marseilles. At the age of 110, she got a Sony Walkman, which she used to listen faithfully to the morning and evening news.

However, her most striking characteristic may have been her lifelong love of physical activity. In her youth, Calment played tennis, fenced, and roller skated. She and her husband hiked in the Alps, and hunted partridge and wild boar in the Provençal hills. She dashed to St. Trophime's every evening until she was 108, and made a daily trek to the cemetery 1 km away where her husband, daughter, and grandson were buried. She is said to have ridden her bicycle until she turned 100. She lived at home alone and climbed the stairs without help until a fall slowed her down at 110. Even after this, she continued to stretch and do calisthenics every morning.

The health rewards of exercise may seem too good to be true. If a pill was advertised as doing what exercise does, you'd write it off as quackery. But the payoff from exercise is real. In clinical trials, exercise did as well as drugs at preventing death in patients recovering from heart attacks or strokes. Exercise has immediate effects. It reduces anxiety and sharpens the mind. People who exercise fall asleep more easily, sleep more deeply, and spend less time lying in bed half-awake before getting up in the morning. Exercise lowers blood pressure, and improves the body's response to insulin. Physical activity also pays dividends after months to years. It improves cardiac fitness, builds muscle, and lifts depression. It reduces all-cause mortality, heart attacks, strokes, type 2 diabetes, high cholesterol, cancer, dementia, and obesity. It also lowers the risk of those scourges of old age, falls and osteoporosis. Perhaps personal trainers save as many lives as physicians.

Exercise extends life by several paths. One of these is rejuvenating blood vessels. Arteries get stiffer with age, leading to high blood pressure, and eventually to heart attacks, strokes, kidney disease, and dementia. This creeping rigidity is related to falling levels of nitric oxide in the lining of arteries. Nitric oxide relaxes muscles in the walls of blood vessels, opening them up and increasing blood flow. (Nitroglycerin pills, or "nitro," reduce the chest pain of coronary disease because they release nitric oxide.) Exercise restores the ability of blood vessels to make nitric oxide. A happy by-product of this vascular alchemy is the healthy glow that comes with exercise.

Another superpower of exercise is its ability to lower blood sugars. Sugary Western diets lead to obesity and diabetes. In the early stages of adult-onset diabetes, also known as pre-diabetes, the body becomes less responsive to insulin, and the pancreas must crank out more and more insulin to restore blood sugars to normal. This phenomenon is known as insulin resistance, and it progresses to full-blown diabetes if unchecked. Exercise turns muscles into glucose-hungry sponges which suck up excess blood sugar. It also decreases body fat and increases muscle mass, restoring insulin sensitivity.

Exercise starves cells of energy and oxygen, and leads to a buildup of heat, acid, and free radicals. Usually, these things are bad. However, the stress of exercise switches on the same life-extending genes that are activated by caloric restriction (this is an example of hormesis, or the beneficial biologic effects of moderate intermittent stress). Exercise turns on genes involved in fixing broken DNA and mopping up free radicals. It also reduces inflammation, boosts the production and repair of mitochondria, and protects telomeres. Athletes have longer telomeres than non-athletes, and active older adults have longer telomeres than their sedentary peers. Exercise also seems to prevent telomere erosion in people with high levels of psychological stress.

Happily, the doses of exercise which prolong life and fight middle-aged dry rot are rather low. The Physical Activity Guidelines for Americans recommend 150 minutes of moderate aerobic activity or 75 minutes of vigorous aerobic activity weekly, or an equivalent mix of both. Adults should also do muscle strengthening workouts of at least moderate intensity twice weekly, such as pushups, situps, or lifting weights. In a cohort of nearly 480,000 adults followed for a median of nine years, Min Zhao and colleagues found that all-cause mortality was 11% lower in those who did the recommended muscle workouts, 29% lower in those who met the guidelines for aerobic exercise, and 40% lower in those who did both, after the usual adjustments for lifestyle factors and chronic health conditions. These results also held up after excluding people with chronic health problems which might have affected their ability to exercise. Weekend warriors, who cram their workouts into one or two days, seem to have the same reduction in all-cause mortality as people who exercise throughout the week.

Moderate and vigorous exercise are defined in terms of METs, which stands for metabolic equivalent of task. One MET is the amount of energy your body uses sitting still. Moderate activity requires three to six METs, and vigorous activity more than six METs.

With moderate activity, you may break a light sweat, and your breathing and heart rates go up a bit, while vigorous activity leads to profuse sweating, heavy breathing, and rapid pulse. From a health perspective, a minute of vigorous activity, such as running, swimming laps, or singles tennis, is equal to two minutes of moderate activity, such as brisk walking, yard work, housework, or doubles tennis. Team sports, such as basketball or soccer, count as vigorous exercise, while cycling can be moderate or vigorous, depending on intensity.

If you use a fitness tracker, such as a Fitbit, Apple Watch, or step-counting smartphone app, how much activity should you shoot for? A sample of 4840 men and women in the National Health and Nutrition Examination Survey wore accelerometers for a week. (An accelerometer, as you'll recall, is the technical name for an activity tracker.) The participants, who had an average age of 57, were followed for the next 10 years. The lowest all-cause mortality was seen in those who did 12,000 steps per day, with no additional survival benefit beyond this point. Step speed did not affect mortality. Sprinters and plodders had similar death rates, as long as they did the same number of daily steps. For older people, lower step counts may be fine. Among nearly 17,000 participants in the Women's Health Study, with an average age of 72, the risk of death hit a plateau at around 7500 steps per day, or somewhat over three miles a day of walking.

Can you exercise too much? While couch potatoes are more likely to die young than gym rats, there may be a modest downside to prolonged high-volume exercise. Atrial fibrillation, an irregular heart rhythm that increases the risk of stroke, may be more common in male endurance athletes. In a meta-analysis, atrial fibrillation was 6% *less* common in men and women who did moderate amounts of exercise, compared to those who were physically inactive. However, men who did high volumes of exercise had the same risk of atrial fibrillation as men who were sedentary. Women who were highly active did not seem to be predisposed to atrial fibrillation, perhaps in keeping with the greater overall resilience of women. In a cohort of over 200,000 Swedish cross-country skiers who completed distance races, an elevated risk of atrial fibrillation was seen in male skiers who entered more races and had fast finishing times. Again, this tendency toward atrial fibrillation was not seen in women, perhaps because men are more liable to develop heart chamber enlargement in response to exercise.

Overtraining may also lead to cardiac fibrosis, or scar tissue on the heart. In a study from Barcelona, radiologists compared heart MRIs of 93 hard-core triathletes to less-active controls. The triathletes had an average age of 36 years, and had trained for at least 12 hours a week for the past five years, while the control subjects did less than three hours of sports and exercise per week. The triathletes had mild cardiac enlargement, a normal response to training known as athlete's heart. But they were also 10 times more likely to have patchy scar tissue where the right ventricle attaches to the septum, the muscular wall that separates the right and left sides of the heart. The long-term significance of this finding is unclear, but it supports the notion that there are diminishing returns with extreme doses of exercise.

CHAPTER 31

State of Nature

Live near trees.

White ash is the Gary Cooper of hardwoods: strong, stolid, blandly handsome. Its stoic tolerance of abuse makes it ideal for axe handles and Louisville Sluggers. It is, or rather was, a common urban tree in the American Midwest. In 2002, forests of white ash started dying off outside of Detroit. The culprit was found to be the emerald ash borer, a rangy iridescent beetle that had somehow found its way over from Asia. Borers lay their eggs in the diamond-shaped crannies of the bark of ash trees. When the eggs hatch, the larvae burrow into the sapwood, creating a network of tunnels that cut off the flow of nutrients and water through the tree.

As the ash borer spread through the Midwest over the next decade, it killed off 100 million mature ash trees. Entire city streets lost their shade trees, leaving them barren and exposed. The borer usually spread from tree to tree, but sometimes it jumped to faraway counties, apparently brought there in loads of firewood. This created a jumbled patchwork of affected and unaffected counties, some with deforestation, some not.

According to one analysis, this loss of tree cover had an unexpected aftershock. Between 2002 and 2007, counties infested with the emerald ash borer had an extra 6,113 deaths from respiratory causes, and 15,080 deaths from cardiovascular causes, compared to counties that were not infested. The excess mortality was more marked in wealthy areas, which tend to have more street trees.

How do trees promote human health? A canopy of urban trees reduces pollution by acting as a gigantic air filter. City air is rife with toxic particulate matter, such as $PM_{2.5}$, which worsens COPD, damages blood vessels, and increases all-cause mortality. In cities with tree cover, significant amounts of $PM_{2.5}$ stick to the waxy surfaces of leaves, to be eventually washed away by rainwater. Leaves also suck up and neutralize gaseous pollutants such as ozone, nitrogen dioxide, and sulfur dioxide, which irritate the lungs. (Some species, such as oaks and sweetgums, are less beneficial, as they give off compounds that promote ozone formation.)

Trees also reduce stress. Time spent in green space lowers heart rate and cortisol levels. In Japan, meandering through forests for better health is known as *shinrin-yoku*, "forest bathing." In a Chinese study, older adults with high blood pressure were randomly assigned to stay either in a hotel in the city of Hangzhou, or a hotel near a large evergreen forest in the country. Both groups ate similar diets, and had similar daily schedules, except that one group spent three hours a day in the city, and the other spent three hours a day in the forest. After one week, the forest group had significantly lower blood pressures and lower levels of the inflammatory cytokine IL-6, compared to the city group.

Numerous studies have shown that living near green space is associated with lower levels of self-reported stress, depression, and anxiety. It has even been shown, in a study from London, that rates of antidepressant prescribing are lower in boroughs with more street trees, even after adjusting for income. One way that green space may bolster mental health is by acting as a social glue, providing places to meet, walk with friends and dogs, play sports, or tend community gardens. In a Dutch study, adults living near green space felt less lonely and reported more social support.

Greater access to green space has been shown to boost mental health. In Philadelphia, researchers identified 541 vacant lots (American cities have a total area of blighted land equal in size to

Switzerland). They grouped nearby neglected lots together, and randomized these clusters to get either conversion to green space, trash cleaning only, or no intervention. In the greening group, garbage, tires, and abandoned cars were removed, the lots were graded, trees and grass were planted, and a low fence was installed, with openings to allow visits. Those who lived near greened lots were less likely to feel depressed and worthless after the intervention, compared to the group with no intervention. The researchers also found that green space even seemed to calm the fabled hostility of Philadelphians. In the poorest neighborhoods, conversion of blighted land to usable green space was associated with significant reductions in gun violence, burglary, public nuisance offenses, and overall crime rates.

Cardiovascular health seems to be better in people who live near green space, perhaps because they are more physically active. In one study, people in the top quartile of neighborhoods for green space were 34% more likely to exercise, compared to those who lived in the bottom quartile. This association was stronger in women and in young adults, and persisted after adjustment for confounders like income.

Your risk of dying also seems to be lower if you live near an abundance of greenery. In one study, the health bonus from having 11 more trees per city block was the equivalent of being 1.4 years younger. A Swiss study and a Canadian study took data from tax records, death registries, and the long-form census, and matched this up with measures of vegetation from satellite imaging. Wealth is an obvious confounder in this kind of study, as moneyed folk tend to prefer tree-lined suburbs, so both studies adjusted for income, air pollution, neighborhood socioeconomic status, and other variables. In the Swiss study, the risk of death was 6% less in those who resided in the 75th percentile of green space (at the higher end of greenness), compared to those at the 25th percentile for green space (toward the lower end of greenness). In the Canadian study, the risk of death was 5% lower in greener communities. While proximity to green space reduced death from a variety of causes, the greatest reductions were in deaths from respiratory disease.

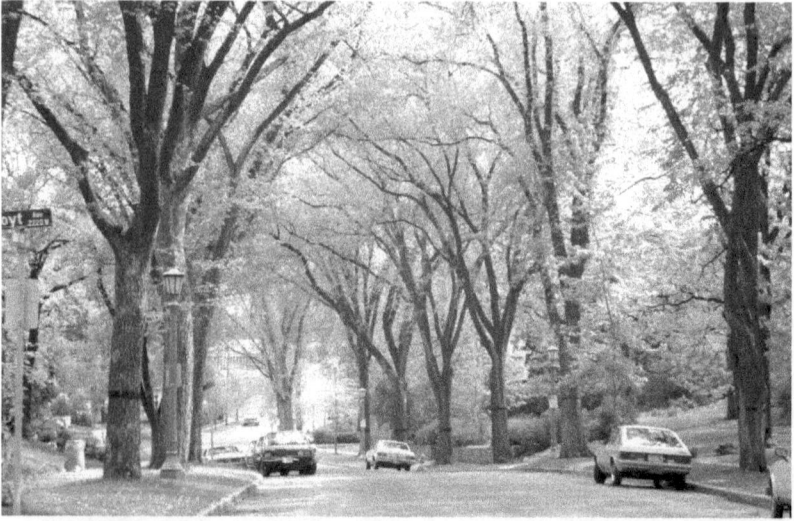

Street lined with American elms. Living in a neighborhood with an abundance of trees is associated with better mental, heart, and lung health. Courtesy of Joseph O'Brien, USDA Forest Service, Bugwood.org.

The importance of green space and trees to human health is likely to grow because of climate change, and a phenomenon known as the urban heat island effect. In the daytime, summer temperatures in cities are around 5°F warmer than the surrounding suburbs. Cities have more waste heat being pumped out from vehicles, machinery, and air conditioners, and fewer trees to give shade and release cooling water vapor. Air stagnates between tall buildings, creating broiling, breezeless urban canyons.

The heat island effect is worse at night, when cities may be 20°F warmer than the suburbs. Concrete, pavement, and brownstone absorb heat during the day, and release it at night, so urban areas never cool down. The heat island effect is predicted to worsen in future, making heat waves more frequent and more severe. City dwellers will be at high risk not only for hyperthermia, but also conditions such as stroke, heart attacks, and kidney failure, which are more common in the setting of dehydration.

CHAPTER 32

Hit Me With Your Best Shot

Get an annual flu shot, get a one-time pneumonia shot when you reach 65, and stay vaccinated against COVID.

In the emergency room at the old Boston City Hospital, I once saw a healthy young woman die from a brain herniation. A herniation is when a bodily organ protrudes into a space where it doesn't belong. It is never good when organs herniate, and when the organ involved is the brain, it is very bad indeed. The day before, the woman got a throbbing headache that wouldn't go away. Bright lights caused agonizing pain. The following morning, she became drowsy and confused, and her family brought her to the hospital. A CT scan revealed that her brain was massively swollen from a fulminant case of meningitis. Because the brain is stuck inside a bone box, that swelling had nowhere to go but down, pressing out through the big opening at the base of the skull called the foramen magnum. The prolapsing brain flattened her medulla, and she stopped breathing and went into cardiac arrest.

The culprit was *Streptococcus pneumoniae*, also known as the pneumococcus. This bacterium is a common cause of pneumonia and meningitis in adults, and was once a prolific killer of both young and old. William Osler, the father of internal medicine, called it "the Captain of the Men of Death." But in a quiet triumph for public health, cases of sepsis, blood infections, and meningitis caused by the pneumococcus have fallen by 90% in American children over the last 20 years. The reason? A new generation of highly effective pneumonia vaccines.

I'm a big fan of vaccination. Because of vaccines, smallpox has been eradicated. Epidemics of paralysis from polio are a thing of the past. Measles, which once killed 6,000 Americans a year, is now a rarity in the United States (though this may change if anti-vaxxers get their way). Compared to many medical treatments, such as a lifetime of pills to control high blood pressure, vaccines need only a minimal commitment of time and energy.

The effectiveness of vaccines may be underestimated by clinical trials involving a relatively small number of people. Vaccines work best when most of the population has received them. If enough people are immune to a given bacteria or virus, it can't gain enough of a foothold to cause an outbreak. Spread of infection then becomes impossible, the state of affairs known as herd immunity. These collateral benefits may be pleasantly surprising. For example, the 90% reduction in serious pneumococcal infections in kids after the introduction of childhood vaccination was accompanied by an unexpected 50% reduction in serious pneumococcal infections in adults. Apparently, a lot of sick grownups with pneumococcal infections had been getting them from kids.

While high vaccination rates help achieve herd immunity, falling ones weaken it. Another example of this comes from Japan. From 1962 to 1987, influenza vaccination was mandatory for Japanese schoolkids. This mandate was relaxed in 1987, and repealed completely in 1994. Childhood vaccination rates against influenza dropped to low levels. Annual mortality from influenza and pneumonia started to go up in adults in 1987, and rose sharply after 1994. (An episode of flu increases the risk of subsequent bacterial pneumonia.) Based on the bump in adult mortality during the phase-out of childhood flu vaccination, it is estimated that 1 adult death had been prevented for every 420 children vaccinated. (At the time, Japan had a larger percentage of households with grandparents and grandchildren living together than most high-income countries.)

Assuming you've had the usual childhood immunizations, which vaccines are most likely to protect you as an adult? The *pneumococcal conjugate vaccine* is a good place to start. It protects against *Streptococcus pneumoniae*, a much-feared cause of pneumonia and meningitis in adults, and the pathogen that led to brain herniation in my patient at Boston City Hospital. A one-time dose of PCV20 (Prevnar 20) is recommended at age 65.

A 2020 review by Fawziah Marra and her colleagues at the University of British Columbia found a 22% reduction in all-cause mortality with adult pneumococcal vaccination. (This review looked at an older version of the pneumococcal vaccine, PPSV23, which is probably a little less effective than PCV20).

Influenza vaccine. Winter may or may not be the season to be jolly, but 'tis certainly the season of excess mortality. In the United States, death rates are 25% higher in the winter. The main cause seems to be enhanced transmission of cold and flu viruses. Low humidity allows viruses to linger in the air, and dries up the mucus layer in the airways that prevents infections. Crowded indoor conditions, as in school classrooms, rev up viral spread. Viruses rip up the lining of the respiratory tract, leading to flares of COPD and asthma, and make it easier for bacteria to get into the lungs and cause pneumonia. If you've ever had full-blown flu, you'll remember how miserable and achy you felt. Influenza fills your body with inflammation, which is a risk factor for acute cardiovascular events. In the week after a bout of flu, the risk of a heart attack is six times higher, and that of stroke eight times higher than normal.

Influenza virus is a tricky sombitch that mutates faster than Zsa Zsa Gabor went through husbands. Because it takes eight months to manufacture and distribute flu vaccine, the strains in the vaccine and those spreading during flu season may not match up exactly. This is why vaccine effectiveness in any given flu season can be as high as 60% and as low as 10%. Even so, there is plenty of evidence that a yearly flu vaccine is the smart choice for health and longevity.

Recent Cochrane Reviews concluded that flu vaccine reduced the risk of influenza by 59% in healthy adults, and by 58% in elderly adults. These studies did not show reductions in all-cause mortality, probably because they weren't large enough to do so. A recent meta-analysis of recent observational studies by Yangyang Cheng and colleagues concluded that older adults who received flu vaccine had a 26% lower risk of cardiovascular events such as heart attacks and stroke, an 18% lower risk of respiratory complications such as pneumonia, and a 43% reduction in all-cause mortality.

Lots of observational studies have shown that flu vaccination is associated with lower mortality. Observational studies use real-world data, in which people decide for themselves whether to get a medical treatment or not, as opposed to a randomized clinical trial, in which the assignment to treatment or placebo is left to chance.

A weakness of observational studies is healthy user bias (or to be more specific, healthy vaccinee bias). That is, the sort of person who goes to the doctor regularly and gets a flu shot every year may differ in many ways from slackers who don't. People who are more conscientious about seeing the doctor may also be more likely to exercise, eat whole foods, and remember to take medications. This could give a false impression of the effectiveness of the flu vaccine. We have some interesting insights into the strength of this effect thanks to Bruce Fireman and his colleagues at Kaiser Permanente, the insurance behemoth that dominates the California health care market. Fireman looked at over 20,000 deaths of older patients over nine flu seasons. He found that patients who got the flu vaccine had lower mortality year-round, not just during flu season, suggesting a major role for healthy user bias. After adjusting for this, they found that the flu vaccine was still associated with a 4.6% reduction in all-cause mortality.

Older adults produce less antibody in response to flu vaccine than young adults. If you are over 65 years old, you should receive either high-dose flu vaccine or adjuvanted flu vaccine, which lead to higher antibody levels and greater protection against flu, compared to standard flu shots.

What about **COVID-19 vaccines**? SARS-CoV-2 is, or at least was, ten times deadlier than influenza. Early in the pandemic, case fatality rates for COVID were estimated to be around 0.8%, compared to the 0.05% case fatality rate of influenza. Since then, death rates have fallen due to better treatment, rising population immunity from vaccinations and infections, and variants which are less lethal, if more contagious. Most COVID deaths occur because of COVID pneumonia and respiratory failure, but COVID kills in other ways. It provokes an inflammatory storm that raises the risk of heart attacks, strokes, and blood clots, even in people that don't need to be admitted to the hospital for pneumonia. Compared to controls, non-hospitalized COVID patients were twice as likely to have a heart attack, and seven times more likely to have a blood clot in the lung (pulmonary embolism).

Real-world data from Hungary strongly suggests that COVID vaccination reduces the risk of death. Using a national database, Hungarian researchers compared the survival of 4 million fully vaccinated adults to 2.4 million completely unvaccinated adults during the third COVID wave in 2021. After adjusting for socioeconomic status and baseline health conditions, they found that, compared to the unvaccinated, recipients of the Moderna mRNA vaccine had a 42% reduction in all-cause mortality, and those who got the Pfizer-BioNTech mRNA vaccine had a 51% reduction in all-cause mortality.

Vaccines haters argue that the best and safest route is "natural immunity," that is, immunity acquired from COVID infection, instead of vaccination. Research by Wangzu Hu and his colleagues at the Indiana University School of Medicine provides evidence that this is a dreadful idea. Using a statewide database, they identified pairs of people with similar age, socioeconomic status, and baseline health conditions who were 30 days out from either COVID-19 infection or a dose of COVID-19 vaccine, and looked at their outcomes over the next several months. (Infections in the first COVID wave, which had a very high mortality, were excluded.) All-cause mortality was 37% higher in the "natural immunity" group, compared to the vaccinated group, even though the natural immunity group was somewhat less likely to get another COVID infection. This suggests that getting COVID if you are unprotected by vaccination has long-term adverse health consequences.

CHAPTER 33

Screen Time

Screening for high blood pressure, high cholesterol, cervical and colon cancer, and HIV disease are the primary care interventions most likely to extend life expectancy.

Disease screening is the notion that doctors can detect diseases early and reliably with safe and inexpensive tests, and that early diagnosis prolongs life and has minimal harms. This is often true. However, sometimes this is merely truthy, a word coined by Stephen Colbert, and defined by him as "[seeming] like truth—the truth we want to exist."

As already discussed, screening and treating *high blood pressure* decreases the risk of heart attacks, strokes, and death. *Statin drugs* were developed to lower blood cholesterol. However, they also reduce heart attacks, strokes, and all-cause mortality in patients with other cardiovascular risk factors, such as hypertension, diabetes, and cigarette smoking. A 2013 Cochrane review found that the use of statins to prevent vascular disease was associated with a 14% reduction in all-cause mortality, as well as lower rates of heart attack and stroke. The American College of Cardiology has an online Atherosclerotic Cardiovascular Disease Risk Estimator to determine if you are likely to benefit from statin treatment. An emerging side effect of statins is an increased risk of type 2 diabetes. This is more common in patients on high doses of statins.

Most studies show that cancer screening lowers the risk of cancer death. However, evidence for reductions in all-cause mortality are weak, and overdiagnosis and underdiagnosis are major problems. Screening is great at catching cancers that grow slowly and gradually. However, some of these indolent cancers might never lead to symptoms, and unnecessary treatment may have serious side effects that could reduce life expectancy. Conversely, many cancers grow too quickly to be picked up on occasional screening tests. These aggressive cancers are usually more lethal.

Let's look at the evidence for and against screening for specific cancers. Screening for *cervical cancer* has an excellent risk-benefit ratio. Pelvic exams to obtain samples for testing are safe (albeit uncomfortable), and early treatment of precancerous lesions is usually curative. Cancer of the uterine cervix was once the leading cause of cancer death in American women, but death rates have plunged in the past 40 years, probably due to widespread screening. About 80% of women in the United States are up to date on their Pap smears, in which cells collected from the cervix are examined for precancerous changes. Cervical specimens may also be screened for infection with high-risk human papillomavirus (HPV) strains. There are about 120 strains of HPV. Some cause common warts and plantar warts. Others are sexually transmitted, and cause genital warts. A handful of these genital HPV strains are carcinogenic, and can lead to cervical, penile, or anal cancers.

In 2000, women in the Osmanabad district of India between the ages of 30 and 59 were randomized to receive either one round of screening for HPV, or no screening at all. This study was judged to be ethical because there was essentially no access to HPV screening in rural India at that time. Of the 131,746 women who were recruited, only eight had previously been screened. After eight years of follow-up, the risk of death from cervical cancer was 35% lower in the women who had either a Pap smear or high-risk HPV testing. All-cause mortality was similar in both screened and unscreened groups, perhaps because the study was not large enough to detect a change from the high background death rate from other causes.

The US Preventive Services Task Force (USPSTF) recommends that women aged 21 to 29 get a Pap smear every three years. Women aged 30 to 65 years should also have a Pap smear every three years; testing every five years for high-risk HPV infection, or a combined Pap smear and high-risk HPV test every five years are acceptable alternatives. Women older than 65 years who are low-risk and have been screened adequately in the past do not require additional testing. The USPSTF gives cervical cancer screening an A grade, meaning a high certainty of substantial net benefit. (Adolescent girls and young women should also get HPV vaccines, which are associated with large reductions in precancerous lesions of the cervix. The HPV vaccine trials were not designed to assess impacts on cervical cancer deaths and all-cause mortality.)

Colon cancer is the third-most common cause of cancer death in the US. The best data to support screening comes from trials of flexible sigmoidoscopy. A "flex sig" is a short scope which only reaches two feet beyond the anus. However, this is long enough to catch 70% of colon cancers and precancers. In one meta-analysis, flex sig was associated with a 2.5% reduction in all-cause mortality, compared to no scope. This translates to an absolute risk reduction of 3 deaths per 1000 persons screened in 11.5 years of follow-up. In the US, flex sig has been largely superseded by colonoscopy, which examines the entire large bowel. Colonoscopy does have risks. Serious bleeding occurs in 0.08% of patients, and bowel perforation in 0.03%, usually when large polyps are removed. Death is rare, but has been reported.

In the Nurses' Health Study and Health Professionals Follow-up Study, cohorts with nearly 89,000 participants followed for 22 years, the risk of dying from colon cancer was 41% lower in those who had a sigmoidoscopy, and 68% lower with colonoscopy, compared to never getting scoped. In a Korean cohort study with over half a million people, colonoscopy in patients ≥45 years was associated with a 29% reduction in all-cause mortality, and a 48% reduction in colon cancer mortality. (Because subjects were not randomly assigned, these studies are also at risk for healthy user bias. People who fuss more about their health and take better care of themselves might be more likely to get scoped.)

The NordICC trial, a randomized trial of colonoscopy from northern Europe that came out in 2022, showed an 18% reduction in colorectal cancer in the colonoscopy group, but failed to show a mortality reduction. This study has been criticized for the relatively brief duration of follow-up and the weirdly low number of colonoscopies performed (of the nearly 85,000 men enrolled in the study, fewer than 12,000 underwent colonoscopy). Other large trials of screening colonoscopy are underway.

For persons at average risk, the USPSTF recommends a colonoscopy every 10 years, starting at age 50, and ending at age 75. The USPSTF gives this recommendation an A grade, meaning a high certainty of substantial net benefit. The risks and benefits after age 75 are less clear, and decisions should be made on an individual basis, depending on a patient's functional status, life expectancy, and desire to be treated if something is found.

The tradeoffs with *breast cancer* screening are more complex. Pap smears and colonoscopies usually lead to cures of precancers, without major harms. However, mammography is prone to overdiagnosis, with greater potential for collateral damage from unnecessary medical care.

Breast cancer rates are 50% higher in the mammography era. This is at least partly due to overdiagnosis. Randomized trials suggest that one in five cancers detected by mammography would progress very slowly, or not at all, if followed without treatment. According to the 2016 USPSTF guidelines, "Even with the [more] conservative estimate of 1 in 8 breast cancer cases being overdiagnosed, for every woman who avoids a death from breast cancer through screening, 2 to 3 women will be treated unnecessarily."

Excess radiation is a particular danger of overdiagnosis. Radiation therapy for breast cancer increases the risk of lung cancer, especially in smokers. For cancers of the left breast, radiotherapy leads to a higher risk of heart attacks, due to spillover of radiation onto the heart.

A 2013 Cochrane review of seven large trials that enrolled over 600,000 women did not find that mammography reduced all-cause mortality, although it was associated with a 19% lower risk of death from breast cancer. A 2016 meta-analysis by Heidi Nelson and colleagues had similar results, with mammography being associated with 22% reduction in the risk of death from breast cancer in women between the ages of 50 and 69. Nelson found no benefit of mammography for women in their 40s or 70s. Nelson's meta-analysis also found no reduction in all-cause mortality.

There are two major explanations for the failure of cancer screening trials to show lower overall rates of death. First, reductions in cancer deaths may be negated by deaths from side effects of treatment. Second, cancer screening may decrease net mortality, but since the absolute number of deaths prevented by screening is fewer than commonly supposed, enormous clinical trials would be required to detect this difference. According to Martin Yaffe and James Mainprize at the University of Toronto, for a mammography trial to show an 18% reduction in deaths from breast cancer, with a corresponding 2% reduction in all-cause mortality, it would need to enroll over a million women, and follow them for at least 10 years. Without such trials, it is impossible to say with certainty whether mammography reduces the overall risk of death in women at average risk for breast cancer.

The 2016 USPSTF guideline gives mammography a B grade, stating that there is moderate certainty of moderate net benefit of mammography every two years in women aged 50 to 74. (This is a downgrade from prior years. The 1996 guideline had given mammography an A grade.) Mammography in women aged 40 to 49 gets a C grade, meaning that the net benefit in this age group is likely to be small. (Note that these guidelines are intended for women at average risk of breast cancer. The benefits of screening are likely to be higher in women at higher risk.)

Lung cancer is the most common cause of cancer death in the United States, with 90% of cases occurring in cigarette smokers. Several high-quality trials have shown that yearly low-dose CT scans, compared to chest x-rays, lead to earlier diagnosis and fewer deaths from lung cancer in current and former smokers. However, all-cause mortality is the same whether smokers are screened with CT scans or regular chest x-rays. Perhaps the CT scan groups had complications from surgery and radiation exposure that offset the survival benefit from lung cancer, or perhaps a larger trial would have been needed to show a drop in all-cause mortality.

The USPSTF recommends annual screening for lung cancer with low-dose CT scans in adults aged 55 to 80 years who have a 30 pack-year smoking history and currently smoke or have quit within the past 15 years. This recommendation gets a B grade.

According to an old saying in medicine, more men die with *prostate cancer* than because of it. The prostate gland makes seminal fluid which nourishes sperm cells, and is thus essential for male fertility. But as men age, the prostate becomes a thoroughgoing nuisance. It slowly enlarges under the influence of testosterone, enfeebling the urinary stream, and gritty debris is trapped within the gland. The prostate becomes a backed-up cesspool of inflammation, in which microscopic islands of cancerous tissue commonly develop. Thankfully, most of these microtumors do not cause problems during life. Among men aged 70-79, unsuspected prostate cancer is found at autopsy in 36% of White Americans, and 51% of Black Americans.

The blood test prostate-specific antigen (PSA) is commonly used as a screening test for early prostate cancer. However, clinical trials suggest that it leads to meddlesome and harmful treatment in men who may never have become ill. In a recent meta-analysis by Dragan Ilic of five randomized controlled trials enrolling over 720,000 men, PSA screening did not prolong life expectancy, and had minimal to no impact on death rates from prostate cancer. Moreover, treatment of early, asymptomatic prostate cancer carries a serious downside. Surgery and radiation for prostate cancer increase the risk of impotence, incontinence, and urinary tract infections. Ilic and his colleagues calculated that for every 1000 men screened for prostate cancer, one would develop urinary sepsis, three would require pads or diapers for urinary incontinence, and 25 would become impotent. Other studies have shown that the risk of death from suicide or heart attack is higher in the months after a new diagnosis of prostate cancer.

PSA screening in men aged 55 to 69 has been given a C grade by the USPSTF, meaning moderate certainty that the net benefit, if any, is likely to be small. PSA screening in men 70 and older gets a D grade, meaning a strong likelihood of no benefit. (Again, these USPSTF recommendations for cancer screening are intended for people at average cancer risk. Those who have strong family histories of cancer, or who carry genes that increase cancer risk, are likely to benefit from more aggressive screening.)

The USPSTF also gives an A grade to *HIV testing*, recommending that all people between the ages of 15 and 65 years should be screened for HIV at least once. Those in high-risk groups, such as men who have sex with men, injection drug users, and people with sexual partners in high-risk groups or of unknown HIV status, should be screened more frequently. There is an abundance of evidence that early treatment of HIV decreases the risk of death.

CHAPTER 34

The Frailty of Our Powers

To prevent falls and frailty, take care of your bones and eyes, mix aerobic, strength, and balance training into your workouts, and be wary of medications that may provoke confusion.

Old age isn't a battle; old age is a massacre.

—Philip Roth, *Everyman*

On March 14, 2007, Kurt Vonnegut was taking his dog for a walk when he tumbled down the steps of his Manhattan brownstone, and landed face-first on the sidewalk below. Though he was still mentally sharp, the 84-year-old writer had been feeling poorly for months. A lifetime of smoking had caught up to him, and he had lost weight and was feeling weak and tired after a bout of bronchitis. Vonnegut was rushed to the hospital and found to have severe brain injuries. He never awoke from a coma, and died four weeks later. As the man himself might have said, so it goes.

As in Vonnegut's case, frailty is often a harbinger of death. Frailty is a syndrome of generalized decline in the elderly, characterized by weight loss, exhaustion, low physical activity, slowness, and weakness. The frail lack vigor, and often restrict their activity because of fear of falls. They may be under siege by a host of chronic medical conditions. But the most crucial piece is loss of reserve. To be frail is to have maxed-out credit cards and an overdrawn bank account, and have to live in a house with a cracked foundation or leaky roof and no way to fix it. The frail have nothing left in case of emergency. Any illness, an episode of pneumonia, a urinary tract infection, even a bad case of the flu, can finish them off, or leave them so weak that they wind up as a permanent resident of a nursing home.

Frailty is hard to reverse once it is established. Let's look at measures to prevent (or at least stave off) frailty, and its most dreaded and potentially life-altering consequence, falling.

Osteoporosis. Low bone mass is an independent predictor of death in older patients. Thirty percent of elderly patients with a hip fracture die in the next 12 months. The US Preventive Services Task Force recommends bone mineral density testing to screen for osteoporosis in all women aged 65 years and over. Women younger than 65 years may benefit from bone mineral density testing if they have multiple risk factors. This may be measured with an online calculator, such as the FRAX® Fracture Risk Assessment Tool. (The benefits of screening in men are not as well established, but some groups recommend screening men over 70 years.) In randomized clinical trials, osteoporosis treatment is associated with an 11% drop in all-cause mortality. There are several effective treatments for osteoporosis. The most commonly prescribed drugs, the bisphosphonates, should not be given beyond five years, as prolonged use may impair the ability of bone to repair wear and tear.

Vitamin D is essential for bone and muscle health. Most of the vitamin D in our bodies is produced in the skin with sun exposure in the summer. Dietary sources of vitamin D are limited, and include fatty fish such as salmon and mackerel, shiitake mushrooms, and dairy products with added vitamin D. Replacing vitamin D in people with very low levels is associated with a small, but significant, decrease in all-cause mortality. Older studies of vitamin D repletion showed reductions in falls and fractures, although the results of more recent studies have been less impressive. Vitamin D supplements are probably most beneficial in patients with low vitamin D levels to start with. If you are over 65 years old, it is probably a good idea to have your 25-hydroxyvitamin D level measured. Low vitamin D levels are very common in housebound elders in wintry climes, such as the frail hospitalized patients I see in Boston. Studies have shown that up to 87% of such patients have vitamin D deficiency. There is no benefit to having levels of vitamin D that are high, as opposed to merely adequate, and some studies have shown worse outcomes in patients with sky-high vitamin D levels.

Vision. Our sense of balance depends partly on our eyesight, and the decline in vision with age increases fall risk. Vision loss may have a gradual onset, and not be recognized until too late. Once you hit the age of 60, you should have an annual visual exam to assess for treatable diseases such as glaucoma, cataracts, and macular degeneration.

Nutrition. Weight loss may be a sign of a serious problem, such as a lurking cancer. But it might also have a benign explanation, such as ill-fitting dentures or side effects of medication. Poor appetite is also caused by isolation, depression, food insecurity from poverty, or a monotonous diet due to impaired ability to shop or cook. Older persons who are losing weight should have a medical evaluation, a consultation with a registered dietitian, and an assessment of social needs. Homebound persons may benefit from elder services and programs such as Meals on Wheels.

Exercise. Exercise is one of the few interventions which has been shown to reduce falls in the elderly in clinical trials. Older adults who are frail, or pre-frail, should exercise two or three times weekly for 45 minutes. In addition to aerobic exercise, which can be as simple as walking or using a stationary bike, sessions should include balance, flexibility, and resistance training. Strength work should focus on the legs, especially the quadriceps, hamstrings, and gluteus muscles, which are critical in transitioning from sitting to standing. Tai chi improves strength, balance, and flexibility, and is associated with a lower risk of falls in the elderly. Classes at a senior center or YMCA offer the added stimulus of social interaction.

Home modifications. Bathrooms are a minefield for frail seniors. An unplanned trip to the toilet at 3 am is as dangerous as leaving the cabin in the woods in a horror movie to investigate those weird noises outside. If you or a loved one suffers from frailty, change the physical environment to reduce the risk of falls. Put automatic night lights in the hallways. Get rid of clutter and obstructions that may lead to falls. Throw away slippery rugs and moldy bathmats. Install easy-grip grab bars to make getting in and out of the bathtub, and on and off the toilet, safer. Consider a raised toilet seat. Put adhesive non-slip strips in the bathtub. Use a shower chair or bath bench, with a handheld shower attachment. Reorganize closets and kitchens so that frequently used items are within easy reach.

Polypharmacy. Elderly patients on multiple medications are at high risk of hospital admission, dementia, and death. In some cases, this may be due to reverse causation. A high burden of diseases that require medication might be the problem, rather than the number of pills. However, try to avoid medicines with a track record of harm in aging patients (see table).

Commonly-used drugs that may harm older patients

Drug class	Typical agents (indication)	Potential harms
Anticholinergics	Amitriptyline (antidepressant), oxybutynin (urinary incontinence), paroxetine (antidepressant)	Delirium, dementia, falls, urinary retention
Antihistamines	Chlorpheniramine, dimenhydrinate, diphenhydramine (allergy and sinus symptoms)	Delirium
Benzodiazepines	Alprazolam (insomnia), diazepam (anxiety)	Falls, delirium, fractures
Fluoroquinolone antibiotics	Ciprofloxacin (urinary tract infection), levofloxacin (pneumonia)	Achilles tendon rupture, aortic aneurysm rupture, *Clostridioides difficile* colitis ("C. diff")
Narcotics	Oxycodone, hydromorphone (acute severe pain)	Aspiration pneumonia, delirium, falls
Non-steroidal anti-inflammatory drugs (NSAIDs)	Ibuprofen, indomethacin, naprosyn (arthritis)	Gastrointestinal bleeding, kidney injury
Proton-pump inhibitors	Esomeprazole, omeprazole, pantoprazole (esophagitis, gastritis)	All-cause mortality, *Clostridioides difficile* colitis, kidney disease, osteoporosis, vitamin B12 deficiency; generally restrict use to 8 weeks or less

CHAPTER 35

Enormous Changes at the Last Minute

There is no clinical evidence yet to support supposed longevity drugs.

I want more life, fucker!

—Rutger Hauer, *Blade Runner*

To recap the book thus far: for a long life, you need to do stuff that may be boring and hard, such as leading a purposeful life, exercising regularly, eating whole foods, and keeping up your social ties. It also helps to be female, affluent, short, and intelligent (think Julia Louis-Dreyfus).

If you bought this book hoping for a quick fix for aging, a royal road to rejuvenation, or magic beans for longevity, you may be feeling a little ripped off. If this is the case, then this chapter is for you! In it, we'll look at some of the more plausible treatments to forestall aging, and the evidence for each. (Please note that the drugs described in this chapter are not ready for prime time. None of them have been scientifically proven to extend life in humans, and many may have serious side effects.)

Rapamycin and other inhibitors of mTOR. In 1964, Georges Nógrády, a microbiologist at the University of Montreal, left the snowdrifts of Quebec for the balmy shores of Easter Island, supposedly to find out why tetanus was so rare there. Rapa Nui, as the island is known to locals, should have been an ideal place to get lockjaw, if one was so inclined. The islanders went shoeless on the rocky ground, and often had cuts on their feet, which would have provided excellent points of entry for tetanus bacteria.

Nógrády divided the island into 67 parcels of one square mile in area, and gathered clumps of earth from each plot. On schlepping his specimens back to Montreal, Nógrády found that his medical mystery had a rather mundane solution. Easter Islanders didn't get tetanus because the bacterium that caused it was nearly absent from their soils. Having no further use for his samples, Nógrády passed them along to researchers at Ayerst Laboratories.

What would a pharmaceutical company want with a pile of Polynesian dirt? For the drug industry, buckets of exotic mud were a potential gold mine. Bacteria and fungi have been fighting an evolutionary arms race for millions of years. Penicillin began as a chemical weapon made by fungi to clear bacteria off their territory. Conversely, the yeast-killing drug nystatin was a poison that bacteria made to kill off their moldy competition. Drugs that we imagine to be the results of elegant experiments are merely the products of brute force testing of vast quantities of earth. *Streptomyces* bacteria were especially prized as prolific producers of lethal compounds, something like a microbial IG Farben. Over 20 drugs have been isolated from different strains of *Streptomyces*, including antibiotics, antifungals, and even antiparasitic and cancer chemotherapy drugs.

Lurking in the dirt from Easter Island was a previously unknown *Streptomyces* species. To the delight of the scientists from Ayerst, this bacterium made a powerful substance that was lethal to fungi. They called this chemical rapamycin, after the island of its origin, Rapa Nui. Rapamycin had other, odder properties. In high doses, it was a powerful immune suppressant. This made rapamycin unsuitable for fighting fungal infections, but attractive as a drug to prevent kidney transplants from being rejected. Another peculiar quality was its ability to prevent cells from multiplying. Cardiologists now keep clogged coronary arteries open with stents that are coated with rapamycin, which stops plaque from regrowing. (Confusingly, when rapamycin is used in clinical medicine, it is known as sirolimus.)

Most impressive of all, rapamycin fooled cells into thinking they were running low on energy, even though there was plenty of fuel around. It did this by interfering with one of the cell's sensing mechanisms for nutrients, the protein called mTOR (mammalian target of rapamycin). This suggested that rapamycin could provide the longevity benefits of calorie restriction, without the discomfort of foregoing food, or the side effects of frailty and bone loss.

Several studies in mice back this up. Giving rapamycin to mice that are 20 months old, the mouse equivalent of 65 human years, extends their median lifespan by 60%. Not only do these mice live longer, but they age more slowly. Compared to their untreated brethren, mice that get rapamycin are more active and flexible, have better memory and cognition, and develop less heart and arterial stiffness. Unfortunately, mice who get rapamycin were also more likely to get cataracts and testicular atrophy. As Connie Mack said, you can't win 'em all.

Studies of rapamycin in other, longer-lived mammals are underway. The Dog Aging Project, which is funded by the National Institute on Aging, is currently studying the effects of rapamycin on canine survival. They are looking for volunteers, if you know of any good boys or girls who would like to stick around as long as possible.

The mTOR protein is a subunit of two larger protein complexes that self-assemble, like combiner robots in *Transformers*. These are known as mTORC1 and mTORC2. These protein complexes have different jobs, and interfering with them with rapamycin has different effects. The life-extending benefits of rapamycin seem to be mainly related to inhibition of mTORC1. Lowering the action of mTORC1 shifts cellular resources away from growth, and into cleanup and maintenance. Cells under the influence of rapamycin gobble up and destroy the damaged proteins and organelles that lead to premature cell death. On the other hand, many of the undesirable side effects of rapamycin, such as high blood sugars, high cholesterol, and insulin resistance, seem to be related to blocking mTORC2.

One strategy that might help to shut down mTORC1, while leaving mTORC2 alone, is to give rapamycin in low or intermittent doses. Another approach is to tinker with the rapamycin molecule itself, creating more selective blockers of mTORC1. Promising rapalogs, or analogues of rapamycin, include drugs such as DL001 and everolimus.

Metformin. Before the modern era, goat's-rue enjoyed a mixed reputation. It was widely detested as a noxious weed that killed sheep and other livestock, who collapsed frothing at the mouth if they ate too much. On the other hand, goat's-rue was one of the few herbal remedies of medieval Europe that seemed to help patients with excessive urination, a cardinal sign of diabetes. In the 1920s, a drug derived from goat's-rue named Synthalin was found to lower blood sugars in diabetics, but it unfortunately led to liver and kidney failure. Plus, it was less effective than the newfangled shot called insulin that a pair of Canadians had recently discovered.

In the 1950s, a new drug named metformin began to be used in Europe to treat diabetes. Metformin was chemically related to Synthalin, but with the advantage of generally not killing people. It did tend to cause a buildup of lactic acid in the blood in patients with advanced kidney disease, which delayed its approval for use in the United States until 1994.

Metformin does many things at a cellular level that could slow aging. It makes cells more sensitive to the action of insulin (as you'll recall, resistance to insulin is common in the old and overweight, and is part of the pro-aging constellation of derangements in the metabolic syndrome). It prevents the liver from producing too much glucose. Perhaps most important, it interferes with energy generation in mitochondria. This dupes cells into thinking that they are undergoing calorie restriction. The misfiring mitochondria send out the same distress signals that are transmitted in actual calorie restriction. The net result is more investment in maintenance. Inflammation is curtailed, free radicals are mopped up more aggressively, and damaged DNA, proteins, organelles, and mitochondria are repaired or replaced. This basic upkeep of the cell extends its lifespan, in the same way that cleaning the roof gutters, getting rid of termites and carpenter ants, and keeping the electrical wiring up to code prolongs the life of your house.

Metformin might also work by a simpler mechanism: weight loss. Metformin is an appetite suppressant. The average person enrolled in a clinical trial of metformin loses 1.1 kg (2.4 lbs). In the Diabetes Prevention Program, patients who got individualized diet and exercise training lost more weight in the short term, but long-term weight loss was more common in those who received metformin.

Metformin has shown inconsistent results in animal studies of life extension. It increases lifespan in flatworms, but not fruit flies. Inbred and short-lived strains of mice live longer when given metformin, but the results are unimpressive in longer-lived and outbred mouse varieties.

In observational studies, metformin treatment has been associated with lower rates of dementia, cancer, and all-cause mortality. However, a Cochrane Reviews meta-analysis of clinical trials did not find a reduction in all-cause mortality in diabetic patients who received metformin.

Metformin is on track to be the first putative anti-aging drug subjected to a large rigorous clinical trial. Led by Nir Barzilai of Albert Einstein Medical College in the Bronx, the TAME study aims to recruit 3000 older adults without diabetes to receive metformin or placebo over a six-year period. Major end-points will include all-cause mortality, dementia, diabetes, cancer, and heart disease. (TAME is a good example of the cringey tradition of contrived acronyms for clinical trials. It stands for Targeting Aging with MEtformin.)

Senolytics. As we've discusssed, some cells are forced to take early retirement because of critical levels of damage to their DNA and telomeres. This prevents them from becoming cancer cells.

Unfortunately, these beat-up cells hang around, in a zombie-like state called cellular senescence. These rogue cells poison their surroundings with inflammation, like a hateful neighbor whose dogs poop in your yard, and who wakes you up on a peaceful Saturday morning with his gas-powered leaf blower. This inflammation damages nearby cells, and they too become senescent. When senile cells are injected into vigorous young mice, a wave of senescence spreads through their bodies like an infection. One month after the transplant, the mice are rodent geriatric cases. Their walking is slowed, their grip is feeble, and they tire easily.

In horror movies, zombies can only be slain by destroying their brains. Zombie cells, on the other hand, are much more vulnerable. To stay alive, they need a steady stream of chemical communications to prevent them from committing suicide. Drugs that kill off these cellular ghouls by interrupting these signals are known as senolytics. (Animal cells somewhat resemble the volcanic lairs of supervillains in James Bond films, in that they are programmed to self-destruct when necessary. As you'll recall, this phenomenon is known as apoptosis.)

In one experiment, when elderly mice were fed a cocktail of two senolytic drugs, *dasatinib* and *quercetin*, it increased their lifespan by 36%. Dasatinib is a chemotherapy agent, used in the treatment of certain leukemias. Quercetin is an antioxidant found in many foods, including onions, capers, hot peppers, apples, asparagus, and berries. A three-day course of dasatinib and quercetin in diabetics with kidney disease reduced the number of senescent cells in fatty tissue, as well as blood levels of inflammatory proteins such as interleukin-6. Three days may not seem like very long, but senolytic drugs will probably need to be given in such brief, intermittent, "hit-and-run" treatments. While senescent cells are usually bad actors, they occasionally turn good. For example, senescence is a necessary part of tissue repair and wound healing, limiting the amount of scar tissue that is produced.

Another polyphenol antioxidant, *fisetin*, is twice as powerful as quercetin in its senolytic activity. Strawberries and apples are rich dietary sources of fisetin. The Mayo Clinic is currently running a study of the effects of fisetin in the prevention of frailty and inflammation in elderly women. The old-timey heart drug *digoxin* is said to have senolytic properties as well. (I am skeptical that it will be shown to have anti-aging benefits, as clinical trials of digoxin in heart disease failed to show reductions in all-cause mortality.)

Acarbose. The complex starches in foods such as rice, potatoes, and bread are made up of long chains of glucose, strung together like lights on a Christmas tree. In the gut, a protein called alpha-glucosidase snips individual glucose molecules off the ends of starch chains, allowing them to be absorbed into the bloodstream. Acarbose, a medicine occasionally used in diabetes, blocks alpha-glucosidase, thus slowing down the absorption of glucose from the bowel. This reduces the spike in blood sugars after eating, which has been implicated as a factor in aging. Acarbose is generally safe, with the major side effect being a socially awkward tendency to gassiness and bloating.

Acarbose extends lifespan in mice. Oddly, this effect is more robust in male mice than females. Male mice given acarbose live 20% longer, while female mice live only 5% longer. Castrated mice do not display this exaggerated longevity in response to acarbose. Perhaps they are too depressed at having been unmanned.

In human studies, acarbose leads to an average weight loss of 0.4 kg, or about one pound. Acarbose has not been associated with reduced all-cause mortality in clinical trials. In a large study which followed 6,500 patients with coronary disease and pre-diabetes for five years, rates of heart attacks, strokes, kidney failure, and death were similar in patients who received acarbose and placebo. (Patients who received acarbose were less likely to develop full-blown diabetes.)

Spermidine. Cloth merchants have long used magnifying glasses to verify the thread counts of fabrics, and avoid getting ripped off by unscrupulous weavers. An 18th-century Dutch draper named Antonie van Leeuwenhoek took this obsession with optics to extremes, grinding ever smaller and more precise lenses, until he accidentally invented the microscope. Leeuwenhoek was the first to describe the appearance of bacteria, red blood cells, and muscle fibers. He also discovered sperm, being careful to specify in his letters to the Royal Society in London that he used semen retrieved from his wife's vagina after lawful coitus, and not obtained through the sin of self-abuse. Leeuwenhoek also noticed that when semen was left at room temperature for several minutes, peculiar crystals began to form.

A German biochemist named Otto Rosenheim spent twenty years studying these deposits, which he called "sperma crystals." Presumably, faced with this stiff challenge, Rosenheim took matters into his own hands, and made frequent sacrifices on the altar of science. He eventually found that these crystals in ejaculate were made up of two different molecules, which he named spermine and spermidine. Together, these polyamines produce semen's pungent aroma.

While spermine may also have health benefits, there is more data for lifespan extension with spermidine. Yeast, fruit flies, and flatworms live longer when their diets are supplemented with spermidine. In wild-type mice, spermidine boosts median lifespan by 10%. Like other geroprotector molecules, spermidine increases the amount of cellular energy invested in infrastructure, getting rid of worn-out proteins and mitochondria, and replacing them with new ones. In animal models, it also lowers blood pressure and enhances immunity.

Spermidine is essential to cellular function, and readers may be relieved to learn that there are other dietary sources of spermidine besides semen. These include wheat germ, peas, lentils, red beans, broccoli, and cauliflower. Aged cheeses, mushrooms, and pine nuts are especially rich in spermidine. (The spermidine content of the Mediterranean diet is high.)

Spermine and spermidine levels generally decline with aging, although centenarians have been found to have polyamine levels similar to those of the middle-aged. High dietary spermidine intake has been associated with a lower risk of death in a prospective observational study. However, a randomized controlled trial of spermidine supplements in older adults with early dementia found that it did not slow down memory loss.

Sirtuin activators. In 2006, sales of red wine surged after reports that resveratrol, a compound found in the skins of grapes and berries, might extend life. If this seemed too good to be true, it probably was. While resveratrol prolongs lifespan in yeast, fruit flies, and flatworms, the data for life extension in mice is inconsistent, and studies in diabetics and other people with metabolic diseases have had disappointing results. (It's easier to extend the lifespan of a short-lived fruit fly than a long-lived human, just as it's easier to make a faster go-kart than a faster Formula 1 car.)

The supposed longevity effect of resveratrol has to do with its ability to turn on sirtuins, a family of proteins that shift resources into DNA repair. Sirtuins bind to a chemical called NAD, or nicotinamide adenine dinucleotide. NAD is like a molecular Venmo which shuttles energy around the cell. It exists in two forms: a high-energy form, NADH, and a low-energy form, NAD+. Sirtuins are switched on by the presence of large amounts of NAD+, an indicator that the cell is stressed and low on energy, and needs to shift into survival mode.

Nicotinamide riboside (NR) and nicotinamide mononucleotide (NMN) are highly touted nutraceuticals that are said to raise NAD+ levels. While benefits have been shown in animal models, there is no convincing evidence for their efficacy in humans at present. One argument against their use is that cells are perfectly capable of making their own NAD+, using either the amino acid tryptophan, the supposed cause of sleepiness after a heavy meal of Thanksgiving turkey, or the essential vitamin niacin.

Growth hormone. A 2007 review of human growth hormone (HGH) treatment in older patients noted that the average patient gained 2.1 kg in muscle mass, while losing a similar amount of fat. However, treatment with HGH was associated with significant harms, including carpal tunnel syndrome, joint pain, leg swelling, and diabetes. Men who took HGH were also prone to develop breast swelling.

Resetting the epigenetic clock: the Yamanaka factors. There is a major theory of aging that we haven't touched on yet: loss of epigenetic information. Cells turn genes on and off by sticking chemical labels on them, a process called epigenetics. Some genes are bedecked with baubles of carbon and hydrogen atoms, known as methyl groups. This methylation is a big NO TRESPASSING sign, a warning to avoid these genes and not transcribe them into proteins.

There are two major reasons why some genes are designated as no-go areas. Stem cells and fetal tissue have very little methylated DNA. In fetal development, as tissues differentiate into kidney cells and heart cells and so on, some genes are turned off with methyl tags. This prevents muscle cells from getting notions and trying to act like brain cells, for example. The other reason is that large chunks of the human genome are not just junk, but destructive junk. We carry around fossil remnants of ancient viruses in our DNA called retrotransposons. If these selfish genes aren't turned off with methyl groups, they can multiply and insert more copies of themselves randomly throughout the genome. This genetic copypasta can damage and inactivate other genes, and even lead to cancer.

As cells age, DNA methylation is one of many things that goes awry. More DNA is methylated in old cells than young cells. Moreover, in old cells, these methyl groups tend to be in the wrong places. DNA that should be shut down is turned on, while access to essential genes is lost, leading to cellular anarchy and misrule. The cell is like a drunken librarian who has shelved books in the wrong stacks, and can't find them anymore. In human studies, the degree of DNA methylation, also known as the epigenetic clock, is a robust predictor of lifespan.

DNA damage makes this problem worse. Imagine a crew of workers that digs up a road to fix a leaky water main, but leaves the gaping hole in the road when they're done. Something similar seems to be happening when cells repair DNA damage. Even if the DNA is repaired correctly, the act of fixing it ages the cell by upsetting its epigenetics.

This was shown in an elegant experiment published in 2023 by Jae-Hyun Yang, David Sinclair, and colleagues. They inserted genes in mice that led to frequent breaks in DNA. These breaks occurred in regions that didn't code for genes, so that any mutations would be essentially harmless. After several months, the mice with the frequent DNA breaks appeared older, compared to control mice. Not only did they have gray hair, muscle weakness, and memory problems, they also had epigenetic changes consistent with premature aging. Even more impressive, Yang and Sinclair claimed to have reversed this excessive DNA methylation with a cocktail of rejuvenation genes, known as Yamanaka factors. Yang and Sinclair wrote that "aging in mammals [is] the equivalent of a software problem, the result of corrupted epigenetic information that can be restored from an existing back-up copy."

The Yamanaka factors have tremendous promise for organ regeneration. Sinclair, working with Yuancheng Lu, had previously reported using them to restore sight in mice with glaucoma. Lu's methods were not for the squeamish. He injected the mice in the eyeballs with a virus carrying a cocktail of Yamanaka factors. This injection made the retinal cells in the back of the eye regress to a younger state, with youthful methylation patterns, and even induced them to sprout new nerve endings. This technique, if safe and effective in humans, might lead not only to recovery of vision, but also reversal of paralysis in patients with spinal cord injuries.

But the use of Yamanaka factors may come with unanticipated risks. María Abad and her colleagues at Spanish National Cancer Research Centre created mice that were programmed to produce four Yamanaka factors on exposure to the antibiotic doxycycline. This successfully wiped out the epigenetic memory of the mouse cells, and restored them to a more younger and more primitive state. Unfortunately, the mice all died of teratomas, hideous tumors which are a gemish of random tissues, such as hair, teeth, fat, muscle, and bone. Oops. There are hopes that a partial reset of adult cells with three of the Yamanaka factors will lead to rejuvenation, without causing cancer. We'll see.

Vampire mice: the parabiosis preparation. Could young blood be a rejuvenating agent? The idea comes straight out of a grim medieval legend, such as Countess Elizabeth Báthory bathing in the blood of her serving girls, or some dystopian sci-fi novel, in which desiccated Boomers cling to life with the help of transfusions from impoverished Millennials. And yet it seems to be true.

The first studies to support this ghoulish idea were done in the 1960s by the brilliant but freaky Clive McCay. McCay, whom you may remember for his work at Cornell showing that half-starved lab rats lived longer, and his claim to have dissolved teeth in Coca-Cola, seems to have specialized in weird science. He sewed pairs of old rats and young rats together, such that they developed a shared blood circulation. (The technical term for this is heterochronic parabiosis.) As you might expect, the rats did not take kindly to this, and had to be sedated for weeks to allow the wounds to heal, and keep them from ripping the sutures apart. McCay found that parabiosis only worked if the rats were closely genetically related. Otherwise, they tended to drop dead a week after the procedure.

If the aging rats survived the surgery, McCay noted that they lived longer than average, and that their tendons were more supple and elastic than those of control animals. McCay was inspired to create even more bonkers Frankenrats, stitching littermates together to create forlorn-looking Siamese triplets and even quadruplets. However, this does not seem to have resulted in additional discoveries of scientific value.

More recently, Saul Villeda at UCSF showed that parabiosis in mice reverses age-related degeneration in the hippocampus, the memory center of the brain. Villeda also showed that geriatric mice did not need to be physically united to their juniors to benefit from their youthful essence. Elderly mice that got plasma from young mice outperformed control oldsters on tests of maze learning and memory. In other studies, plasma from young mice also seemed to improve function and healing in old muscle, liver, kidney, and bone. Conversely, old blood worsened the performance of mitochondria and muscle in young mice.

You probably don't need to sew yourself to your little brother in the hopes of taking advantage of his youthful blood, as cell biologists believe they are close to identifying these anti-aging and pro-aging factors. Candidate anti-aging proteins in blood from young mice include CCL3, CCL4, VEGF, SPARCL1, and TIMP2, while possible pro-aging proteins in blood from old mice include β-2-microglobulin and IL-6 (which, as you'll recall, promotes senescence).

CHAPTER 36

Last Things

You will not live forever. Make your preferences about end-of-life care known beforehand.

Dying is such a long tiresome business.

—Samuel Beckett, "From an Abandoned Work"

We're all on the way out. Act accordingly.

—Jack Nicholson, *The Departed*

Everlasting life was not your destiny.

—*The Epic of Gilgamesh*

Despite buying this book, and religiously abiding by its precepts, you yield at last to nature, and become old and frail. Since the death of your partner two years ago, you feel lonely, eat less, and struggle to keep up with the housework and finances. Your memory and judgment are fading. You recently lost several thousand dollars to a telephone scammer, and voluntarily gave up your driver's license after a fender bender in which you were at fault. Your daughter Constance has been trying for months to get you to sell your home and move to assisted living. You stubbornly refuse, though deep down you know this would be for the best.

When you fail to answer the phone one morning, you are brought to hospital, and found to have a massive stroke that has paralyzed your right side and robbed you of the power of speech. Things go badly. You develop an infection from a urinary catheter, and drift in and out of delirium. Furthermore, the stroke has affected your swallowing. You aspirate into your lungs when you eat and drink, and pneumonia sets in.

Your well-meaning but scattered son Junior, who has spent the past several years in Baja California surfing and sampling the local pharmaceuticals, is now at your bedside, insisting you are a "fighter" who would want everything possible done to keep you alive. You once told Constance that you would not want to go on a ventilator, or get artificial feeding, if you had little chance of living on your own again. Unfortunately, there is no written record of your wishes, and you never designated someone to make medical decisions for you, if you were too sick to make them yourself.

When your breathing fails, the medical team feels obliged to put a breathing tube into your lungs and connect you to a ventilator. Your final weeks of life are spent in intensive care in stupor and pain, with a tracheostomy tube in your throat, a feeding tube in your nose, a central catheter in your jugular vein, a catheter in the radial artery in your wrist to monitor your faltering blood pressure, a catheter in your bladder, and a rectal tube to divert stool away from the bedsores that you've developed.

Stories such as this are all too common in the United States. In surveys, more than 80% of Americans say they want to avoid high-intensity care at the end of life. But many get it anyway, because they left no record of their treatment preferences in the event of critical illness. In the absence of clear guidance to limit care, the default mode in American medicine is to do everything to prolong the duration of life, with little regard to its quality.

The major way to protect yourself against medical care you don't want is an ***advance directive.*** This is a legal document that guides your medical care when you are unable to do so. It may either set limits on treatment, or assign a person to serve as your proxy for if you are incapacitated.

A *living will* (or advance decision, in the UK) directs doctors to forgo or stop life-sustaining treatments in patients who are terminally ill. Living wills are useful, but have limitations. For example, it may not be clear whether a patient's condition is terminal. Also, the term living will is something of a misnomer. It may not be legally binding, depending on how it is worded and where you live.

A *do-not-resuscitate order*, or DNR, indicates that you would never want chest compressions or high-voltage electric shocks if your heart stopped. A *do-not-intubate order*, or DNI, means that you would never want to go on a ventilator. (In the UK, DNR and DNI orders are referred to as DNACPR orders, for "do not attempt cardiopulmonary resuscitation.")

Physician orders for life-sustaining treatment (POLST), also known as medical orders for life-sustaining treatment (MOLST), cover a broad range of scenarios in the chronically ill. For example, in addition to establishing whether or not you want CPR or intubation, they might also address antibiotics, intravenous fluids, a feeding tube, intensive care, dialysis for kidney failure, or whether you'd even want to be admitted to the hospital at all.

A *power of attorney for health care* assigns someone to be your health care proxy. This person, typically a spouse, adult child, or close friend, makes your medical decisions when you cannot. You should designate one person to serve as your primary health care proxy, and another as a backup or alternate health care proxy. It is a bad idea to appoint two equal health care proxies, as they may violently disagree.

A health care power of attorney is probably the most important advance directive. Many goals of care discussions do not involve clear terminal illness and medical futility, and nuanced decision making is required. You should pick a health care proxy who understands your values, and your attitudes towards illness and disability. Are you part of the minority of people who would want to stay alive at any cost? Are you so fiercely independent that you'd be miserable if you had to depend on others for daily care? Or would your quality of life be fine so long as you could spend time with friends and family, despite significant physical or mental impairments?

Your health care proxy should also be someone who sees you regularly, and has a realistic sense of how you were doing before you wound up in the hospital. This is important because your baseline status is predictive of outcome. If you were previously active and independent before becoming critically ill, your chances for recovery are much better than those of someone was already suffering from frailty and dementia.

If you have a high burden of chronic disease, or a terminal illness, you are likely to benefit from seeing a specialist in *palliative care*. A common misconception about palliative care is that it hastens death. This is not true. In a meta-analysis of trials in patients with life-threatening illness, those who were treated by palliative care specialists, in addition to receiving usual care, lived as long as patients who received usual care alone, with a better quality of life.

Palliative care may even *prolong* survival in patients with aggressive cancers. In a randomized, controlled trial in patients with lung cancer that had spread to other organs, patients who were seen early by palliative care had a higher quality of life, were less likely to be depressed or to receive futile care and lived about three months longer than those who were not.

Summary

1. Damage to DNA and telomeres is a major driver of aging.

2. The body shuts down cells with too much DNA damage. This protects against cancer, but contributes to aging.

3. Cells in the human body have a finite number of times they can divide, known as the Hayflick limit. In the short term, this protects against cancer, but in the long term may lead to a vicious cycle of accelerated aging.

4. Human lifespan, which is long relative to most animals, is limited by our ability to maintain the integrity of our DNA.

5. Being tall is associated with a higher risk of cancer death. This risk tends to be balanced out by the higher socioeconomic status of tall people.

6. That which nourishes us also destroys us. When we burn food through the chemical process of oxidation, free radicals are produced, which make our mitochondria age and break down.

7. Protein misfolding is a mechanism of aging that is especially harmful to the brain. It may drive the progression of Alzheimer's and other dementias.

8. If you want to live longer, be a woman. If you can't be a woman, then try not to be a violent, reckless jerk.

9. Calorie restriction extends the life of lab animals by activating genes that shunt energy into DNA repair and cellular maintenance. However, this may not extend human life span, and could have serious side effects such as osteoporosis and frailty.

10. Moderate your salt intake by avoiding processed food and fast food, and eating potassium-rich fruits and vegetables.

11. Red meat gets a lot of bad press, but processed red meat should get most of the blame. Avoid processed red meats such as ham, bacon, hot dogs, sausages, and deli meat.

12. Temper tantrums and a bad attitude can kill you.

13. Avoid smoke, especially cigarette smoke.

14. Promiscuous use of dietary supplements may be associated with serious harm, including death.

15. Avoid ultraprocessed foods.

16. Avoid drinks and foods with added sugars.

17. Stick to less than seven drinks per week, preferably red wine.

18. Avoid having a firearm in your home, especially a handgun.

19. For longer life, get off your ass.

20. Cultivate your social networks.

21. Don't be poor.

22. Get your blood pressure under control.

23. Maintain a healthy weight with physical activity and a diet of whole foods.

24. A high-fiber diet reduces the risk of obesity and metabolic syndrome.

25. Conscientious people live longer.

26. Stable marriages and partnerships prolong lifespan. This is true for both sexes, but especially so for men.

27. Have a reason to get out of bed in the morning.

28. Moderate amounts of coffee and tea are safe and may prolong life.

29. Stave off dementia by staying physically, socially, and intellectually active.

30. Do 150 minutes of moderate aerobic activity, or 75 minutes of vigorous aerobic activity, every week.

31. Live near trees.

32. Get an annual flu shot, get a one-time pneumonia shot when you reach 65, and stay vaccinated against COVID.

33. Screening for high blood pressure, high cholesterol, cervical and colon cancer, and HIV disease are the primary care interventions most likely to extend life expectancy.

34. To prevent falls and frailty, take care of your bones and eyes, mix aerobic, strength, and balance training into your workouts, and be wary of medications that may provoke confusion.

35. There is no current clinical evidence to support supposed longevity drugs.

36. You will not live forever. Make your preferences about end-of-life care known beforehand.

References

1. Time Out of Joint

Gilford H. On a condition of mixed premature and immature development. Med Chir Trans 1897;80:17-46.

Gilford H. Progeria: a form of senilism. Practitioner 1904;17:188-217.

Gilford H. Disorders of Post-Natal Growth and Development. London: Adlard and Son, 1911.

Kudlow BA, Kennedy BK, Monnat RJ Jr. Werner and Hutchinson- Gilford progeria syndromes. Nat Rev Mol Cell Biol 2007;8:394-404.

Maynard S, Fang EF, Scheibye-Knudsen M, et al. DNA damage, DNA repair, aging, and neurodegeneration. Cold Spring Harb Perspect Med 2015;5(10):a025130.

Pray L. DNA replication and causes of mutation. Nature Education 2008;1(1):214.

2. This Cell Will Self-Destruct in Five Seconds

Cohen D. The canine transmissible venereal tumor: a unique result of tumor progression. Adv Cancer Res 1985;43:75-112.

Jolie A. My medical choice. New York Times. May 14, 2013:A25.

Lipman R et al. Genetic loci that influence cause of death in a heterogeneous mouse stock. J Gerontol A Biol Sci Med Sci 2004;59:977-83.

Mohanty PK, Arunbabu KP, Aziz T, et al. Transient weakening of Earth's magnetic shield probed by a cosmic ray burst. Phys Rev Lett 2016; 117(17):171101.

Nowaczyk NR, Arz HW, Frank U, et al. Dynamics of the Laschamp geomagnetic excursion from Black Sea sediments. Earth Planet Sci Lett 2012;54:351-2.

Ostrander GK, Cheng KC, Wolf JC, Wolfe MJ. Shark cartilage, cancer and the growing threat of pseudoscience. Cancer Res 2004;64:8485-91.

Rothschild BM, Tanke DH, Helbling M 2nd, Martin LD. Epidemiologic study of tumors in dinosaurs. Naturwissenschaften 2003;90:495-500.

3. Clocks

Bodnar AG et al. Extension of life-span by introduction of telomerase into normal human cells. Science 1998;279:349-52.

Carrel A. The immortality of animal tissues and its significance. Can Med Assoc J 1928;18:327-9.

Friedman DM. The immortalists: Charles Lindbergh, Dr. Alexis Carrel, and their daring quest to live forever. New York: HarperCollins, 2007.

Goldstein S. Studies on age-related disease in cultured skin fibroblasts. J Invest Dermatol 1979;73:19-23.

Hayflick L. A brief history of the mortality and immortality of cultured cells. Keio J Med 1998;47:174-82.

Reggiani AH. Alexis Carrel, the unknown: eugenics and population research under Vichy. Fr Hist Stud 2002;25:331-56.

Seluanov A et al. Telomerase activity coevolves with body mass not lifespan. Aging Cell. 2007;6:45–52.

Witkowski JA. Dr. Carrel's immortal cells. Med Hist 1980:24:129-42.

4. Planned Obsolescence

Colchero F, Rau R, Jones OR, et al. The emergence of longevous populations. Proc Natl Acad Sci USA 2016;113:E7681-E7690.

Dong X, Milholland B, Vijg J. Evidence for a limit to human lifespan. Nature 2016;538:257-9.

Keane M, Semeiks J, Webb AE, et al. Insights into the evolution of longevity from the bowhead whale genome. Cell Rep 2015;10:112-22.

Kirkwood T. Time of Our Lives. Oxford: Oxford University Press, 1999.

Moore LT, McEvoy B, Cape E, Simms K, Bradley DG. A Y-chromosome signature of hegemony in Gaelic Ireland. Am J Hum Genet 2005;78:334-8.

Quesada V, Freitas-Rodríguez S, Miller J, et al. Giant tortoise genomes provide insights into longevity and age-related disease. Nat Ecol Evol 2019;3:87–95.

Trinkaus E. Late Pleistocene adult mortality patterns and modern human establishment. Proc Natl Acad Sci USA 2011;108:1267-71.

Zerjal T, Xue Y, Bertorelle G, et al. The genetic legacy of the Mongols. Am J Hum Genet 2003;72:717-21.

5. Size Matters

He Q, Morris BJ, Grove JS, et al. Shorter men live longer: association of height with longevity and FOXO3 genotype in American men of Japanese ancestry. PLoS One 2014;9:e94385.

Ihira H, Sawada N, Iwasaki M, et al. Adult height and all-cause and cause-specific mortality in the Japan Public Health Center-based Prospective Study (JPHC). PLoS One. 2018;13(5):e0197164.

Kabat GC, Anderson ML, Heo M, et al. Adult stature and risk of cancer at different anatomic sites in a cohort of postmenopausal women. Cancer Epidemiol Biomarkers Prev 2013;22:1353-63.

Lai FY, Nath M, Hamby SE, et al. Adult height and risk of 50 diseases: a combined epidemiological and genetic analysis. BMC Med 2018;16(1):187.

Lemez S, Wattie N, Baker J. Do "big guys" really die younger? An examination of height and lifespan in former professional basketball players. PLoS One 2017;12:e0185617.

Sawada N, Wark PA, Merritt MA, et al. The association between adult attained height and sitting height with mortality in the European Prospective Investigation into Cancer and Nutrition (EPIC). PLoS One 2017;12:e0173117.

Sohn K. Now, the taller die earlier: the curse of cancer. J Gerontol A Biol Sci Med Sci 2016;71:713-9.

Sutter NB, Bustamante CD, Chase K, et al. A single IGF1 allele is a major determinant of small size in dogs. Science 2007;316:112–5.

Tyrrell J, Jones SE, Beaumont R, et al. Height, body mass index, and socioeconomic status: mendelian randomisation study in UK Biobank. BMJ. 2016;352:i582.

Vazquez JM, Sulak M, Chigurupati S, Lynch VJ. A zombie LIF gene in elephants is upregulated by TP53 to induce apoptosis in response to DNA damage. Cell Rep 2018;24:1765-76.

Zöller B, Ji J, Sundquist J, Sundquist K. Body height and incident risk of venous thromboembolism. Circ Cardiovasc Genet 2017;10:e001651.

6. Burning Man

Gladyshev VN. The free radical theory of aging is dead. Long live the damage theory! Antioxid Redox Signal 2014;20:727-731.

Liguori I, Russo G, Curcio F, et al. Oxidative stress, aging, and diseases. Clin Interv Aging 2018;13:757-72.

Lyons TW, Reinhard CT, Planavsky NJ. The rise of oxygen in Earth's early ocean and atmosphere. Nature 2014;506:307-15.

Kasting JF. When methane made climate. Sci Am 2004;291(1):78-85.

Kopp RE, Kirschvink JL, Hilburn IA, Nash CZ. The Paleoproterozoic snowball Earth: a climate disaster triggered by the evolution of oxygenic photosynthesis. Proc Natl Acad Sci USA 2005;102:11131-6.

Raz N, Daugherty AM. Pathways to brain aging and their modifiers. Gerontology 2018;64:49-57.

7. Human Origami

Coles LS, Young RD. Supercentenarians and transthyretin amyloidosis: the next frontier of human life extension. Prev Med 2012;54 Suppl:S9-11.

Hartl FU. Protein misfolding diseases. Annu Rev Biochem 2017;86:21-26.

Hipp MS, Kasturi P, Hartl FU. The proteostasis network and its decline in ageing. Nat Rev Mol Cell Biol 2019;20:421-435.

Klaips CL, Jayaraj GG, Hartl FU. Pathways of cellular proteostasis in aging and disease. J Cell Biol 2018;217:51-63.

Soto C, Pritzkow S. Protein misfolding, aggregation, and conformational strains in neurodegenerative diseases Nat Neurosci 2018;21:1332-40.

Trigo D, Nadais A, da Cruz e Silva OAB. Unravelling protein aggregation as an ageing related process or a neuropathological response. Ageing Res Rev 2019;51:67-77.

8. The Weaker Sex

Austad SN. Sex differences in longevity and aging. In: Masuro EJ, Austad SN, eds. Handbook of the Biology of Aging, 7th ed. London: Elsevier, 2011.

Becofsky KM, Shook RP, Sui X, et al. Influence of the source of social support and size of social network on all-cause mortality. Mayo Clin Proc 2015;90:895-902.

Freedman VA, Wolf DA, Spillman BC. Disability-free life expectancy over

30 years: a growing female disadvantage in the US population. Am J Public Health 2016;106:1079-85.

Holt-Lunstad J, Smith TB, Layton JB. Social relationships and mortality risk: a meta-analytic review. PLoS Med 2010;7:e1000316.

Marais GAB, Gaillard JM, Vieira C, et al. Sex gap in aging and longevity: can sex chromosomes play a role? Biol Sex Differ 2018;9:33.

McCurdy SA. Epidemiology of disaster. The Donner Party (1846-1847). West J Med 1994;160:338-42.

Min KJ, Lee CK, Park HN. The lifespan of Korean eunuchs. Curr Biol 2012;22:R792-3.

Mondal D, Galloway TS, Bailey TC, Mathews F. Elevated risk of stillbirth in males: systematic review and meta-analysis of more than 30 million births. BMC Med. 2014;12:220.

Stuckey M. The Donner Party and the rhetoric of Western expansion. Rhet Pub Affairs 2010; 14:229-260.

World Health Organization. World Health Statistics 2016: Monitoring health for the SDGs. Geneva: WHO Press, 2016.

Yang YC, McClintock MK, Kozloski M, Li T. Social isolation and adult mortality: the role of chronic inflammation and sex differences. J Health Soc Behav 2013;54:183-203.

Zarulli V, Jones JAB, Oksuzyan A, et al. Women live longer than men even during severe famines and epidemics. Proc Natl Acad Sci USA 2018;115:E832-E840.

Zhu M, Zhao S, Coben JH, Smith GS. Why more male pedestrians die in vehicle-pedestrian collisions than female pedestrians: a decompositional analysis. Inj Prev 2012;19:227-31.

9. The Hunger Artist

Anton T. The Longevity Seekers: Science, Business, and the Fountain of Youth. Chicago: University of Chicago Press, 2013.

Carlson AJ, Hoelzel F. Apparent prolongation of the life span of rats by intermittent fasting. J Nutr 1946;31:363-75.

Friedman DB, Johnson TE. A mutation in the age-1 gene in Caenorhabditis elegans lengthens life and reduces hermaphrodite fertility. Genetics 1988;118:75-86.

Gruman G. A History of Ideas About the Prolongation of Life. New York: Springer, 2003.

Huisman MH, Seelen M, van Doormaal PT, et al. Effect of presymptomatic body mass index and consumption of fat and alcohol on amyotrophic lateral sclerosis. JAMA Neurol 2015;72:1155-62.

Jenkins NL, McColl G, Lithgow GJ. Fitness cost of extended lifespan in Caenorhabditis elegans. Proc Biol Sci 2004;271:2523-6.

Johnson TE. Increased life-span of age-1 mutants in Caenorhabditis elegans and lower Gompertz rate of aging. Science 1990;249:908-12.

Klass MR. A method for the isolation of longevity mutants in the nematode Caenorhabditis elegans and initial results. Mech Ageing Dev 1983;22:279-86.

Kristan DM. Calorie restriction and susceptibility to intact pathogens. Age (Dordr) 2008;30:147–56.

Lassinger BK, Kwak C, Walford RL, Jankovic J. Atypical parkinsonism and motor neuron syndrome in a Biosphere 2 participant: a possible complication of chronic hypoxia and carbon monoxide toxicity? Mov Disord 2004;19:465-9.

Mariosa D, Beard JD, Umbach DM, et al. Body mass index and amyotrophic lateral sclerosis: a study of US military veterans. Am J Epidemiol 2017;185:362-371.

Mattison JA, Colman RJ, Beasley T, et al. Caloric restriction improves health and survival of rhesus monkeys. Nat Commun 2017;8:14063.

Mattison JA, Roth GS, Beasley TM, et al. Impact of caloric restriction on health and survival in rhesus monkeys from the NIA study. Nature 2012;489:318–321.

Mattson MP, Cutler RG, Camandola S. Energy intake and amyotrophic lateral sclerosis. Neuromolecular Med 2007;9:17-20.

Maugh TH. Roy Walford, 79: eccentric UCLA scientist touted food restriction. Los Angeles Times, May 1, 2004.

McDonald RB, Ramsey JJ. Honoring Clive McCay and 75 years of calorie restriction research. J Nutr 2010;140:1205-10.

O'Reilly ÉJ, Wang H, Weisskopf MG, et al. Premorbid body mass index and risk of amyotrophic lateral sclerosis. Amyotroph Lateral Scler Frontotemporal Degener 2012;14:205-11.

Park HW. Longevity, aging, and caloric restriction: Clive Maine McCay and the construction of a multidisciplinary research program. Hist Stud Nat Sci 2010;40:79-124.

Poynter J. The Human Experiment: Two Years and Twenty Minutes Inside Biosphere 2. New York: Basic Books, 2009.

Ravussin E, Redman LM, Rochon J, et al. A 2-year randomized controlled trial of human caloric restriction: feasibility and effects on predictors of health span and longevity. J Gerontol A Biol Sci Med Sci 2015;70:1097-104.

Reider R. Dreaming the Biosphere. Albuquerque: University of New Mexico Press, 2010.

Vaughan KL, Kaiser T, Peaden R, et al. Caloric restriction study design limitations in rodent and nonhuman primate studies. J Gerontol A Biol Sci Med Sci 2017;73:48–53.

Villareal DT, Fontana L, Weiss EP, et al. Bone mineral density response to caloric restriction-induced weight loss or exercise-induced weight loss: a randomized controlled trial. Arch Intern Med 2006;166:2502-10.

Villareal DT, Fontana L, Das SK, et al. Effect of two-year caloric restriction on bone metabolism and bone mineral density in non-obese younger adults. J Bone Miner Res 2015;31:40-51.

Walford RL, Mock D, MacCallum T, Laseter JL. Physiologic changes in humans subjected to severe, selective calorie restriction for two years in biosphere 2: health, aging, and toxicological perspectives. Toxicol Sci 1999;52(2 Suppl):61-5.

Walford RL, Mock D, Verdery R, MacCallum T. Calorie restriction in biosphere 2: alterations in physiologic, hematologic, hormonal, and biochemical parameters in humans restricted for a 2-year period. J Gerontol A Biol Sci Med Sci 2002;57(6):B211-24.

Weindruch R, Walford RL, Fligiel S, Guthrie D. The retardation of aging in mice by dietary restriction: longevity, cancer, immunity and lifetime energy intake. J Nutr 1986;116:641-54.

10. So Salty

Cogswell ME, Mugavero K, Bowman BA, Frieden TR. Dietary sodium and cardiovascular disease risk—measurement matters. N Engl J Med 2016;375:580-6.

Graudal NA, Hubeck-Graudal T, Jurgens G. Effects of low sodium diet versus high sodium diet on blood pressure, renin, aldosterone, catecholamines, cholesterol, and triglyceride. Cochrane Database Syst Rev 2017;4:CD004022.

Graudal N, Jürgens G, Baslund B, Alderman MH. Compared with usual sodium intake, low- and excessive-sodium diets are associated with increased mortality: a meta-analysis. Am J Hypertens 2014;27:1129-37.

Institute of Medicine. Sodium Intake in Populations: Assessment of Evidence. Washington, DC: National Academies Press, 2013.

Judd SE, Aaron KJ, Letter AJ, et al. High sodium:potassium intake ratio increases the risk for all-cause mortality: the REasons for Geographic And
Racial Differences in Stroke (REGARDS) study. J Nutr Sci 2013;2:e13.

Kurlansky M. Salt: A World History. New York: Walker and Company, 2002.

Messerli FH, Hofstetter L, Syrogiannouli L, et al. Sodium intake, life expectancy, and all-cause mortality. Eur Heart J 2021;42:2103-12.

Mozaffarian D, Fahimi S, Singh GM, et al. Global sodium consumption and
death from cardiovascular causes. N Engl J Med 2014;371:624-34.

O'Donnell M, Mente A, Rangarajan S, et al. Urinary sodium and potassium excretion, mortality, and cardiovascular events. N Engl J Med
2014;371:612-23.

O'Donnell M, Mente A, Rangarajan S, et al. Joint association of urinary sodium and potassium excretion with cardiovascular events and mortality. BMJ 2019;364:l772.

Okayama A, Okuda N, Miura K, et al. Dietary sodium-to-potassium ratio as
a risk factor for stroke, cardiovascular disease and all-cause mortality in
Japan: the NIPPON DATA80 cohort study. BMJ Open 2016;6:e011632.

Powles J, Fahimi S, Micha R, et al. Global, regional and national sodium intakes in 1990 and 2010: a systematic analysis of 24 h urinary sodium excretion and dietary surveys worldwide. BMJ Open 2013;3(12):e003733.

Satou R, Penrose H, Navar LG. Inflammation as a regulator of the renin-angiotensin system and blood pressure. Curr Hypertens Rep
2018;20(12):100.

SPEX CertiPrep. Analysis of gourmet salts for the presence of heavy metals.
Retrieved from: https://www.spexcertiprep.com/knowledge-base/files/
AppNote_GourmetSalts.pdf

Weller O. First salt making in Europe: an overview from Neolithic times.
Documenta Praehistorica 2015;42:185-96.

11. Red Meat Rhetoric

Abbasi J. TMAO and heart disease: the new red meat risk? JAMA 2019;
321:2149-51.

Cao Y, Strate LL, Keeley BR, et al. Meat intake and risk of diverticulitis among men. Gut. 2018;67:466–472.

Diallo A, Deschasaux M, Latino-Martel P, et al. Red and processed meat intake and cancer risk: Results from the prospective NutriNet-Santé cohort study. Int J Cancer 2018;142:230-7.

Eshel G, Shepon A, Makov T, Milo R. Land, irrigation water, greenhouse gas, and reactive nitrogen burdens of meat, eggs, and dairy production in the United States. Proc Natl Acad Sci USA 2014;111:11996-2001.

Etemadi A, Sinha R, Ward MH, et al. Mortality from different causes associated with meat, heme iron, nitrates, and nitrites in the NIH-AARP Diet and Health Study. BMJ 2017;357:j1957.

Heianza Y, Ma W, Manson JE, et al. Gut microbiota metabolites and risk of major adverse cardiovascular disease events and death: a systematic review and meta-analysis of prospective studies. J Am Heart Assoc 2017;6(7). pii: e004947.

Hooda J, Shah A, Zhang L. Heme, an essential nutrient from dietary proteins, critically impacts diverse physiological and pathological processes. Nutrients 2014;6:1080–1102.

Ioannidis JP. Implausible results in human nutrition research. BMJ 2013; 347:f6698.

Khambadkone SG, Cordner ZA, Dickerson F, et al. Nitrated meat products are associated with mania in humans and altered behavior and brain gene expression in rats. Mol Psychiatry. 2018 Jul 18. doi: 10.1038/s41380-018-0105-6.

Koeth RA, Wang Z, Levison BS, et al. Intestinal microbiota metabolism of L-carnitine, a nutrient in red meat, promotes atherosclerosis. Nat Med 2013;19:576–85.

McFarlin BK, Venable AS, Henning AL, et al. Natural cocoa consumption: potential to reduce atherogenic factors? J Nutr Biochem 2015;26:626-32.

Micha R, Wallace SK, Mozaffarian D. Red and processed meat consumption and risk of incident coronary heart disease, stroke, and diabetes mellitus: a systematic review and meta-analysis. Circulation 2010;121:2271-83.

Nielsen TB, Würtz AML, Tjønneland A, Overvad K, Dahm CC. Substitution of unprocessed and processed red meat with poultry or fish and total and cause-specific mortality. Br J Nutr 2022;127:563-9.

Schoenfeld JD, Ioannidis JP. Is everything we eat associated with cancer? A systematic cookbook review. Am J Clin Nutr 2013;97:127-34.

Trotter WR. A Frozen Hell: The Russo-Finnish Winter War of 1939-1940. Chapel Hill: Algonquin Books of Chapel Hill, 1991.

van den Brandt PA. Red meat, processed meat, and other dietary protein sources and risk of overall and cause-specific mortality in The Netherlands Cohort Study. Eur J Epidemiol 2019;34:351-369.

Wang X, Lin X, Ouyang YY, et al. Red and processed meat consumption and mortality: dose-response meta-analysis of prospective cohort studies. Public Health Nutr 2016;19:893-905.

Yan S, Gan Y, Song X, et al. Association between refrigerator use and the risk of gastric cancer. PLoS One 2018;13(8):e0203120.

Zink KD, Lieberman DE. Impact of meat and Lower Palaeolithic food processing techniques on chewing in humans. Nature 2016;531:500-3.

12. Anger Management

Barefoot JC, Larsen S, von der Lieth L, Schroll M. Hostility, incidence of acute myocardial infarction, and mortality in a sample of older Danish men and women. Am J Epidemiol 1995;142:477–484.

Coccaro EF, Lee R, Coussons-Read M. Elevated plasma inflammatory markers in individuals with intermittent explosive disorder and correlation with aggression in humans. JAMA Psychiatry 2014;71:158-65.

Everson SA, Kauhanen J, Kaplan GA, et al. Hostility and increased risk of mortality and acute myocardial infarction: the mediating role of behavioral risk factors. Am J Epidemiol 1997;146:142–52.

Kim ES, VanderWeele TJ. Mediators of the association between religious service attendance and mortality. Am J Epidemiol 2019;188:96-101.

Klabbers G, Bosma H, van den Akker M, et al. Cognitive hostility predicts all-cause mortality irrespective of behavioural risk at late middle and older age. Eur J Public Health 2013;23:701-5.

Lemogne C, Nabi H, Zins M, et al. Hostility may explain the association between depressive mood and mortality: evidence from the French GAZEL cohort study. Psychother Psychosom 2010;79:164-71.

Mostofsky E, Maclure M, Tofler GH, et al. Relation of outbursts of anger and risk of acute myocardial infarction. Am J Cardiol 2013;112:343-8.

Mostofsky E, Penner EA, Mittleman MA. Outbursts of anger as a trigger of acute cardiovascular events: a systematic review and meta-analysis. Eur Heart J 2014;35:1404-10.

Thom NJ, O'Connor PJ, Clementz BA, Dishman RK. Acute exercise prevents angry mood induction but does not change angry emotions. Med Sci Sports Exerc 2019;51:1451-9.

Williams JE, Nieto FJ, Sanford CP, Tyroler HA. Effects of an angry temperament on coronary heart disease risk. Am J Epidemiol 2001;154:230-5.

Williams R. North Korea's "Dear Leader" Kim Jong-il died in fit of rage over dam that had sprung a leak. Independent. December 31, 2012.

13. Filthie Smoake

Brandt AM. The Cigarette Century. New York: Basic Books, 2007.

Cakmak S, Hebbern C, Vanos J, et al. Exposure to traffic and mortality risk in the 1991-2011 Canadian Census Health and Environment Cohort (CanCHEC). Environ Int 2019;124:16-24.

Di Q, Wang Y, Zanobetti A, et al. Air pollution and mortality in the Medicare population. N Engl J Med 2017;376:2513-22.

Hamanaka RB, Mutlu GM. Particulate matter air pollution: effects on the cardiovascular system. Front Endocrinol (Lausanne) 2018;9:680.

Hoek G, Krishnan RM, Beelen R, et al. Long-term air pollution exposure and cardio-respiratory mortality. Environ Health 2013;12:43.

Jbaily A, Zhou X, Liu J et al. Air pollution exposure disparities across US population and income groups. Nature 2022;601:228–33.

Kumar P, Druckman A, Gallagher J, et al. The nexus between air pollution, green infrastructure and human health. Environ Int 2019;133(Pt A):105181.

Lefler JS, Higbee JD, Burnett RT, et al. Air pollution and mortality in a large, representative U.S. cohort: multiple-pollutant analyses, and spatial and temporal decompositions. Environ Health 2019;18(1):101.

Li P, Zhao J, Gong C, et al. Association between individual PM2.5 exposure and DNA damage in traffic policemen. J Occup Environ Med 2014;56:e98-e101.

Liu C, Chen R, Sera F, et al. Ambient particulate air pollution and daily mortality in 652 cities. N Engl J Med 2019;381:705-15.

Jha P, Ramasundarahettige C, Landsman V, et al. 21st-century hazards of smoking and benefits of cessation in the United States. N Engl J Med 2013;368:341-50.

Orru H, Ebi KL, Forsberg B. The interplay of climate change and air pollution on health. Curr Environ Health Rep 2017;4:504-513.

Pearl R. Tobacco smoking and longevity. Science 1938;87:216-7.

Pope CA 3rd, Rodermund DL, Gee MM. Mortality effects of a copper smelter strike and reduced ambient sulfate particulate matter air pollution. Environ Health Perspect 2007;115:679-83.

Rich DQ, Kipen HM, Huang W, et al. Association between changes in air pollution levels during the Beijing Olympics and biomarkers of inflammation and thrombosis in healthy young adults. JAMA 2012;307:2068-78.

Rich DQ, Liu K, Zhang J, et al. Differences in birth weight associated with the 2008 Beijing Olympics air pollution reduction. Environ Health Perspect 2015;123:880-7.

Wei Y, Wang Y, Di Q, et al. Short term exposure to fine particulate matter and hospital admission risks and costs in the Medicare population. BMJ 2019;367:l6258.

14. Supplemental Discipline

Balaji S, Chempakam B. Toxicity prediction of compounds from turmeric (Curcuma longa L). Food Chem Toxicol 2010;48:2951-9.

Bjelakovic G, Nikolova D, Gluud LL, et al. Antioxidant supplements for prevention of mortality in healthy participants and patients with various diseases. Cochrane Database Syst Rev 2012 Mar 14;(3):CD007176.

Denham BE. Dietary supplements--regulatory issues and implications for public health. JAMA 2011;306:428-9.

Geller AI, Shehab N, Weidle NJ, et al. Emergency department visits for adverse events related to dietary supplements. N Engl J Med 2015;373:1531-40.

Hudson A, Lopez E, Almalki AJ, et al. A review of the toxicity of compounds found in herbal dietary supplements. Planta Med 2018;84:613-26.

Lukefahr AL, McEvoy S, Alfafara C, Funk JL. Drug-induced autoimmune hepatitis associated with turmeric dietary supplement use. BMJ Case Rep 2018 Sep 10. pii: bcr-2018-224611.

Omenn GS. Chemoprevention of lung cancers: lessons from CARET, the beta-carotene and retinol efficacy trial, and prospects for the future. Eur J Cancer Prev 2007;16:184-91.

Or F, Kim Y, Simms J, Austin SB. Taking stock of dietary supplements' harmful effects on children, adolescents, and young adults. J Adolesc Health 2019;65:455–61.

Roy-Lachapelle A, Solliec M, Bouchard MF, Sauvé S. Detection of cyanotoxins in algae dietary supplements. Toxins (Basel) 2017 Feb 25;9(3).

Tucker J, Fischer T, Upjohn L, Mazzera D, Kumar M. Unapproved pharmaceutical ingredients included in dietary supplements associated with US Food and Drug Administration warnings. JAMA Netw Open 2018;1(6):e183337.

Wong A, Ngu DY, Dan LA, et al. Detection of antibiotic resistance in probiotics of dietary supplements. Nutr J 2015;14:95.

15. Lost in the Supermarket

Baraldi LG, Martinez Steele E, Canella DS, Monteiro CA. Consumption of ultra-processed foods and associated sociodemographic factors in the USA between 2007 and 2012. BMJ Open 2018;8:e020574.

Blanco-Rojo R, Sandoval-Insausti H, López-Garcia E, et al. Consumption of ultra-processed foods and mortality: a national prospective cohort in Spain. Mayo Clin Proc 2019;94:2178-88.

Chang AR, Lazo M, Appel LJ, et al. High dietary phosphorus intake is associated with all-cause mortality: results from NHANES III. Am J Clin Nutr 2014;99:320-7.

Cohen A. The Lord Justice hath ruled: Pringles are potato chips. New York Times, May 31, 2009.

Darmon N, Drewnowski A. Contribution of food prices and diet cost to socioeconomic disparities in diet quality and health. Nutr Rev 2015;73:643-60.

Fardet A. Minimally processed foods are more satiating and less hyperglycemic than ultra-processed foods: a preliminary study with 98 ready-to-eat foods. Food Funct 2016;7:2338-46.

Hall KD, Ayuketah A, Brychta R, et al. Ultra-processed diets cause excess calorie intake and weight gain: an inpatient randomized controlled trial of ad libitum food intake. Cell Metab 2019;30:67-77.e3.

Harrison R, Warburton V, Lux A, et al. Blindness caused by a junk food diet. Ann Intern Med 2019;171:859-61.

Hoch T, Kreitz S, Gaffling S, Pischetsrieder M, Hess A. Fat/carbohydrate ratio but not energy density determines snack food intake and activates brain reward areas. Sci Rep 2015;5:10041.

Juul F, Martinez-Steele E, Parekh N, et al. Ultra-processed food consumption and excess weight among US adults. Br J Nutr 2018;120:90-100.

Kim H, Hu EA, Rebholz CM. Ultra-processed food intake and mortality in the USA: results from the Third National Health and Nutrition Examination Survey (NHANES III, 1988-1994). Public Health Nutr 2019;22:1777-85.

Li Z, Yang X, Yang J, et al. The cohort study on prediction of incidence of all-cause mortality by metabolic syndrome. PLoS One 2016;11 (5):e0154990.

Martínez Steele E, Juul F, Neri D, et al. Dietary share of ultra-processed foods and metabolic syndrome in the US adult population. Prev Med 2019;125:40-48.

Monteiro CA, Cannon G, Levy RB, et al. Ultra-processed foods: what they are and how to identify them. Public Health Nutr 2019;22:936-41.

Monteiro CA, Moubarac JC, Cannon G, et al. Ultra-processed products are becoming dominant in the global food system. Obes Rev 2013;14 Suppl 2:21-8.

Rico-Campà A, Martínez-González MA, Alvarez-Alvarez I, et al. Association between consumption of ultra-processed foods and all cause mortality: SUN prospective cohort study. BMJ. 2019;365:l1949.

Ritz E, Hahn K, Ketteler M, et al. Phosphate additives in food--a health risk. Dtsch Arztebl Int 2012;109:49–55.

Schnabel L, Buscail C, Sabate JM, et al. Association between ultra-processed food consumption and functional gastrointestinal disorders. Am J Gastroenterol 2018;113:1217-28.

Srour B, Fezeu LK, Kesse-Guyot E, et al. Ultraprocessed food consumption and risk of type 2 diabetes among participants of the NutriNet-Santé prospective cohort. JAMA Intern Med 2020;180:283-291.

Volkow ND, Wise RA. How can drug addiction help us understand obesity? Nat Neurosci 2005;8:555-60.

Warner GR, Flaws JA. Bisphenol A and phthalates: how environmental chemicals are reshaping toxicology. Toxicol Sci 2018;166:246–9.

16. Children of the Corn

Collin LJ, Judd S, Safford M, Vaccarino V, Welsh JA. Association of sugary beverage consumption with mortality risk in US adults. JAMA Netw Open 2019;2:e193121.

DiNicolantonio JJ. Increase in the intake of refined carbohydrates and sugar may have led to the health decline of the Greenland Eskimos. Open Heart 2016;3:e000444.

DiNicolantonio JJ, O'Keefe J. Markedly increased intake of refined carbohydrates and sugar is associated with the rise of coronary heart disease and diabetes among the Alaskan Inuit. Open Heart 2017;4:e000673.

Klein AV, Kiat H. The mechanisms underlying fructose-induced hypertension: a review. J Hypertens 2015;33:912–20.

Kratzer JT, Lanaspa MA, Murphy MN, et al. Evolutionary history and metabolic insights of ancient mammalian uricases. Proc Natl Acad Sci USA 2014;111:3763-8.

Lowette K, Roosen L, Tack J, Vanden Berghe P. Effects of high-fructose diets on central appetite signaling and cognitive function. Front Nutr 2015;2:5.

Malik VS, Li Y, Pan A, De Koning L, et al. Long-term consumption of sugar-sweetened and artificially sweetened beverages and risk of mortality in US adults. Circulation 2019;139:2113-25.

Monnard CR, Grasser EK. Cardiovascular responses to sugar-sweetened beverages in humans. Adv Nutr 2018;9:70-7.

Mullee A, Romaguera D, Pearson-Stuttard J, et al. Association between soft drink consumption and mortality in 10 European countries. JAMA Intern Med 2019;179:1479-90.

Page KA, Chan O, Arora J, et al. Effects of fructose vs glucose on regional cerebral blood flow in brain regions involved with appetite and reward pathways. JAMA 2013;309:63-70.

Ramne S, Alves Dias J, González-Padilla E, et al. Association between added sugar intake and mortality is nonlinear and dependent on sugar source in 2 Swedish population-based prospective cohorts. Am J Clin Nutr 2019;109:411-23.

Schaeffer O. Medical observations and problems in the Canadian Arctic. II. Can Med Assoc J 1959;81:386-93.

Schaeffer O. Eskimos (Inuit). In: Trowell HC, Burkitt DP, eds. Western Diseases: Their Emergence and Prevention. Cambridge, MA: Harvard University Press, 1981.

Shan Z, Rehm CD, Rogers G, et al. Trends in dietary carbohydrate, protein, and fat intake and diet quality among US adults, 1999-2016. JAMA 2019;322:1178-87.

Tasevska N, Park Y, Jiao L, et al. Sugars and risk of mortality in the NIH-AARP Diet and Health Study. Am J Clin Nutr 2014;99:1077-88.

Varley K, Bjerga A. America's corn syrup habit could fill New Jersey. Bloomberg, December 20, 2017.

Yang Q, Zhang Z, Gregg EW, et al. Added sugar intake and cardiovascular diseases mortality among US adults. JAMA Intern Med 2014;174:516-24.

17. Hold My Beer

Boniface S, Shelton N. How is alcohol consumption affected if we account for under-reporting? A hypothetical scenario. Eur J Public Health 2013;23:1076-81.

Costanzo S, Di Castelnuovo A, Donati MB, et al. Wine, beer or spirit drinking in relation to fatal and non-fatal cardiovascular events: a meta-analysis. Eur J Epidemiol 2011;26:833-50.

Gepner Y, Golan R, Harman-Boehm I, et al. Effects of initiating moderate alcohol intake on cardiometabolic risk in adults with type 2 diabetes: a 2-year randomized, controlled trial. Ann Intern Med 2015;163:569-79.

Goulden R. Moderate alcohol consumption is not associated with reduced all-cause mortality. Am J Med 2016;129:180-6.

Huang J, Wang X, Zhang Y. Specific types of alcoholic beverage consumption and risk of type 2 diabetes: A systematic review and meta-analysis. J Diabetes Investig 2017;8:56-68.

Kunzmann AT, Coleman HG, Huang WY, Berndt SI. The association of lifetime alcohol use with mortality and cancer risk in older adults. PLoS Med 2018;15:e1002585.

LoConte NK, Brewster AM, Kaur JS, et al. Alcohol and cancer: a statement of the American Society of Clinical Oncology. J Clin Oncol 2018;36:83-93.

Morgagni G. The Seats and Causes of Diseases: Investigated by Anatomy. Vol. 2. Boston: Wells and Lilly, 1824.

Mukamal KJ, Maclure M, Muller JE, Mittleman MA. Binge drinking and mortality after acute myocardial infarction. Circulation 2005;112:3839–45.

Naimi TS, Brown DW, Brewer RD, et al. Cardiovascular risk factors and confounders among nondrinking and moderate-drinking U.S. adults. Am J Prev Med 2005;28:369–373.

Rehm J, Taylor B, Mohapatra S, et al. Alcohol as a risk factor for liver cirrhosis: a systematic review and meta-analysis. Drug Alcohol Rev 2010;29:437–45.

Rehm J, Roerecke M. Reduction of drinking in problem drinkers and all-cause mortality. Alcohol Alcohol 2013;48:509-13.

Stahre M, Roeber J, Kanny D, et al. Contribution of excessive alcohol consumption to deaths and years of potential life lost in the United States. Prev Chronic Dis 2014;11:130293.

Stockwell T, Zhao J, Panwar S, et al. Do "moderate" drinkers have reduced mortality risk? J Stud Alcohol Drugs 2016;77:185–98.

Wood AM, Kaptoge S, Butterworth AS, et al. Risk thresholds for alcohol consumption: combined analysis of individual-participant data for 599 912 current drinkers in 83 prospective studies. Lancet 2018;391:1513–23.

18. Trigger Warning

Clarke RV, Jones PR. Suicide and increased availability of handguns in the United States. Soc Sci Med 1989;28:805-9.

Conner A, Azrael D, Miller M. Suicide case-fatality rates in the United States, 2007 to 2014. Ann Intern Med 2019;171:885-95.

Dahlberg LL, Ikeda RM, Kresnow MJ. Guns in the home and risk of a violent death in the home. Am J Epidemiol 2004;160:929-36.

Drexler M. Guns and suicide: the hidden toll. Harv Public Health Spring 2013:24-35.

Grassel KM, Wintemute GJ, Wright MA, Romero MP. Association between handgun purchase and mortality from firearm injury. Inj Prev 2003;9:48-52.

Hedegaard H, Curtin SC, Warner M. Suicide mortality in the United States, 1999-2017. NCHS Data Brief 2018;(330):1-8.

Hemenway D. Comparing gun-owning vs non-owning households in terms of firearm and non-firearm suicide and suicide attempts. Prev Med 2019;119:14-6.

Hemenway D, Miller M. Association of rates of household handgun ownership, lifetime major depression, and serious suicidal thoughts with rates of suicide across US census regions. Inj Prev 2002;8:313-6.

Kellermann AL, Reay DT. Protection or peril? An analysis of firearm-related deaths in the home. N Engl J Med 1986;314:1557-60.

Kellermann AL, Rivara FP, Rushforth NB, et al. Gun ownership as a risk factor for homicide in the home. N Engl J Med 1993;329:1084-91.

Kellermann AL, Rivara FP, Somes G, et al. Suicide in the home in relation to gun ownership. N Engl J Med 1992;327:467-72.

Kim H, Kim B, Kim SH, et al. Classification of attempted suicide by cluster analysis: a study of 888 suicide attempters presenting to the emergency department. J Affect Disord 2018;235:184-90.

Knopov A, Sherman RJ, Raifman JR, et al. Household gun ownership and youth suicide rates at the state level, 2005-2015. Am J Prev Med 2019;56:335-342.

Kposowa A, Hamilton D, Wang K. Impact of firearm availability and gun regulation on state suicide rates. Suicide Life Threat Behav 2016;46:678-96.

Naghavi M; Global Burden of Disease Self-Harm Collaborators. Global, regional, and national burden of suicide mortality 1990 to 2016. BMJ 2019;364:l94.

Owens D, Horrocks J, House A. Fatal and non-fatal repetition of self-harm: systematic review. Brit J Psychiatry 2002;181:193-9.

Prickett KC, Gutierrez C, Deb S. Family firearm ownership and firearm-related mortality among young children: 1976-2016. Pediatrics 2019;143(2). pii: e20181171.

Remembering Ryan. Vermont Cynic, December 1, 2008.

Turecki G, Brent DA. Suicide and suicidal behaviour. Lancet 2016;387 (10024):1227-39.

Wintemute GJ, Teret SP, Kraus JF, Wright MW. The choice of weapons in firearm suicides. Am J Public Health 1988;78:824-6.

Zalsman G, Hawton K, Wasserman D, et al. Suicide prevention strategies revisited: 10-year systematic review. Lancet Psychiatry 2016;3:646-59.

19. Sitting Ducks

Chau JY, Grunseit AC, Chey T, et al. Daily sitting time and all-cause mortality: a meta-analysis. PLoS One. 2013 Nov 13;8(11):e80000.

Dempsey PC, Larsen RN, Dunstan DW, et al. Sitting less and moving more: implications for hypertension. Hypertension 2018;72:1037-1046.

Dempsey PC, Sacre JW, Larsen RN, et al. Interrupting prolonged sitting with brief bouts of light walking or simple resistance activities reduces resting blood pressure and plasma noradrenaline in type 2 diabetes. J Hypertens 2016;34:2376-82.

Diaz KM, Howard VJ, Hutto B, et al. Patterns of sedentary behavior and mortality in U.S. middle-aged and older adults. Ann Intern Med 2017;167:465-75.

Ekelund U, Steene-Johannessen J, Brown WJ, et al. Does physical activity attenuate, or even eliminate, the detrimental association of sitting time with mortality? Lancet 2016;388:1302-10.

Ensrud KE, Blackwell TL, Cauley JA, et al. Objective measures of activity level and mortality in older men. J Am Geriatr Soc 2014;62:2079-87.

Harris JL, Bargh JA, Brownell KD. Priming effects of television food advertising on eating behavior. Health Psychol 2009;28:404-13

Katzmarzyk PT, Church TS, Craig CL, Bouchard C. Sitting time and mortality from all causes, cardiovascular disease, and cancer. Med Sci Sports Exerc 2009;41:998-1005.

Koster A, Caserotti P, Patel KV, et al. Association of sedentary time with mortality independent of moderate to vigorous physical activity. PLoS One 2012;7(6):e37696.

Kuper S. The man who invented exercise. Financial Times, September 11, 2009.

Morishima T, Restaino RM, Walsh LK, et al. Prolonged sitting-induced leg endothelial dysfunction is prevented by fidgeting. Am J Physiol Heart Circ Physiol 2016;311:H177-82.

Morris JN, Heady JA, Raffle PA, et al. Coronary heart-disease and physical activity of work. Lancet 1953;262:1053-57, 1111-20.

Safdar A, Hamadeh MJ, Kaczor JJ, et al. Aberrant mitochondrial homeostasis in the skeletal muscle of sedentary older adults. PLoS One 2010;5(5):e10778.

Stamatakis E, Gale J, Bauman A, et al. Sitting time, physical activity, and risk of mortality in adults. J Am Coll Cardiol 2019;73:2062-72.

van der Ploeg HP, Chey T, et al. Standing time and all-cause mortality in a large cohort of Australian adults. Prev Med 2014;69:187-91.

Wijndaele K, Brage S, Besson H, et al. Television viewing and incident cardiovascular disease: prospective associations and mediation analysis in the EPIC Norfolk Study. PLoS One 2011;6(5):e20058.

Wijndaele K, Sharp SJ, Wareham NJ, Brage S. Mortality risk reductions from substituting screen time by discretionary activities. Med Sci Sports Exerc 2017;49:1111-9.

20. So Lonesome I Could Die

Buettner D. The Blue Zones. Washington: National Geographic Society, 2008.

Cacioppo JT, Fowler JH, Christakis NA. Alone in the crowd: the structure and spread of loneliness in a large social network. J Pers Soc Psychol 2009;97:977-91.

Chan YC, Suzuki M, Yamamoto S. Dietary, anthropometric, hematological and biochemical assessment of the nutritional status of centenarians and elderly people in Okinawa, Japan. J Am Coll Nutr 1997;16:229-35.

Cohen S, Doyle WJ, Skoner DP, et al. Social ties and susceptibility to the common cold. JAMA 1997;277:1940-4.

Das A. Loneliness does (not) have cardiometabolic effects: a longitudinal study of older adults in two countries. Soc Sci Med 2019;223:104-12.

Deiana L, Ferrucci L, Pes GM, et al. AKEntAnnos. The Sardinia Study of Extreme Longevity. Aging (Milano) 1999;11:142-9.

Freedman A, Nicolle J. Social isolation and loneliness: the new geriatric giants. Can Fam Physician 2020;66:176-82.

Hajek A, König HH. How do cat owners, dog owners and individuals without pets differ in terms of psychosocial outcomes among individuals in old age without a partner? Aging Ment Health. 2019;1-7.

Harlow HF, Dodsworth RO, Harlow MK. Total social isolation in monkeys. Proc Natl Acad Sci USA 1965;54:90-7.

Harlow H, Harlow M. Social deprivation in monkeys. Sci Am 1962; 207(5):136-50.

Haycock DB. Mortal coil: a short history of living longer. New Haven: Yale University Press, 2008.

Henriksen RE, Nilsen RM, Strandberg RB. Loneliness as a risk factor for metabolic syndrome: results from the HUNT study. J Epidemiol Community Health 2019;73:941-946.

Holt-Lunstad J, Smith TB, Baker M, Harris T, Stephenson D. Loneliness and social isolation as risk factors for mortality: a meta-analytic review. Perspect Psychol Sci 2015;10:227-37.

Larrabee Sonderlund A, Thilsing T, Sondergaard J. Should social disconnectedness be included in primary-care screening for cardiometabolic disease? A systematic review of the relationship between everyday stress, social connectedness, and allostatic load. PLoS One 2019;14(12):e0226717.

Lindsay EK, Young S, Brown KW, et al. Mindfulness training reduces loneliness and increases social contact in a randomized controlled trial. Proc Natl Acad Sci USA 2019;116:3488–93.

Mazess RB, Forman SH. Longevity and age exaggeration in Vilcabamba, Ecuador. J Gerontol 1979;34:94-8.

Pes GM, Tognotti E, Poulain M, Chambre D, Dore MP. Why were Sardinians the shortest Europeans? A journey through genes, infections, nutrition, and sex. Am J Phys Anthropol 2017;163:3-13.

Poulain M, Pes GM, Grasland C, et al. Identification of a geographic area characterized by extreme longevity in the Sardinia island: the AKEA study. Exp Gerontol 2004;39:1423-9.

Rico-Uribe LA, Caballero FF, Martín-María N, et al. Association of loneliness with all-cause mortality: A meta-analysis. PLoS One 2018; 13(1):e0190033.

Schrempft S, Jackowska M, Hamer M, Steptoe A. Associations between social isolation, loneliness, and objective physical activity in older men and women. BMC Public Health 2019;19:74.

Smith KJ, Gavey S, Riddell NE, et al. The association between loneliness, social isolation and inflammation: a systematic review and meta-analysis. Neurosci Biobehav Rev 2020;112:519-41.

Steptoe A, Fancourt D. Leading a meaningful life at older ages and its relationship with social engagement, prosperity, health, biology, and time use. Proc Natl Acad Sci USA 2019;116:1207-12.

Taylor SE, Klein LC, Lewis BP, et al. Biobehavioral responses to stress in females: tend-and-befriend, not fight-or-flight. Psychol Rev 2000;107: 411–29.

Valtorta NK, Kanaan M, Gilbody S, et al. Loneliness and social isolation as risk factors for coronary heart disease and stroke: systematic review and meta-analysis of longitudinal observational studies. Heart 2016; 102:1009-16.

Vella-Burrows T, Pickard A, Wilson L, et al. 'Dance to Health': an evaluation of health, social and dance interest outcomes of a dance programme for the prevention of falls. Arts Health 2019 Sep 6:1-15.

21. The Rich Are Different

Barboza Solís C, Fantin R, Castagné R, et al. Mediating pathways between parental socio-economic position and allostatic load in mid-life: Findings from the 1958 British birth cohort. Soc Sci Med 2016;165:19-27.

Boylan JM, Cundiff JM, Matthews KA. Socioeconomic status and cardiovascular responses to standardized stressors. Psychosom Med 2018;80:278–93.

Brunner EJ, Marmot MG, Nanchahal K, et al. Social inequality in coronary risk: central obesity and the metabolic syndrome. Evidence from the Whitehall II study. Diabetologia 1997;40:1341–9.

Bunker J. Medicine Matters After All: Measuring the Benefits of Medical Care, a Healthy Lifestyle, and a Just Social Environment. London: Nuffield Trust, 2001.

Castagné R, Kelly-Irving M, Campanella G, et al. Biological marks of early-life socioeconomic experience is detected in the adult inflammatory transcriptome. Sci Rep 2016;6:38705.

Chae DH, Wang Y, Martz CD, et al. Racial discrimination and telomere shortening among African Americans. Health Psychol 2020;39:209-219.

Chetty R, Stepner M, Abraham S et al. The association between income and life expectancy in the United States, 2001–2014. JAMA 2016;315:1750–66.

Cutler DM. Life and death in Norway and the United States. JAMA 2019;321: 1877–9.

Dimsdale JE, Hackett TP, Hutter AM Jr, et al. Type A personality and extent of coronary atherosclerosis. Am J Cardiol 1978;42:583–6.

Gump BB, Matthews KA. Are vacations good for your health? The 9-year mortality experience after the multiple risk factor intervention trial. Psychosom Med 2000;62:608-12.

Jones A. After I lived in Norway, America felt backward. The Nation, January 28, 2016.

Kalkhoran S, Berkowitz SA, Rigotti NA, Baggett TP. Financial strain, quit attempts, and smoking abstinence among U.S. adult smokers. Am J Prev Med 2018;55:80-8.

Kaplan JR, Manuck SB. Status, stress, and atherosclerosis: the role of environment and individual behavior. Ann N Y Acad Sci 1999;896:145-61.

Kinge JM, Modalsli JH, Øverland S, et al. Association of household income with life expectancy and cause-specific mortality in Norway, 2005-2015. JAMA 2019;321:1916-25.

Kivimäki M, Batty GD, Pentti J, et al. Association between socioeconomic status and the development of mental and physical health conditions in adulthood: a multi-cohort study. Lancet Public Health 2020;5:e140-9.

Kunz-Ebrecht SR, Kirschbaum C, Marmot M, Steptoe A. Differences in cortisol awakening response on work days and weekends in women and men from the Whitehall II cohort. Psychoneuroendocrinology 2004;29:516-28.

Marmot M. The Status Syndrome: How Social Standing Affects Our Health and Longevity. New York: Times Books, 2004.

Marmot M. The health gap: doctors and the social determinants of health. Scand J Public Health 2017;45:686-693.

Marmot MG, Adelstein AM, Robinson N, Rose GA. Changing social-class distribution of heart disease. Br Med J 1978;2(6145):1109-12.

Marmot M, Allen J, Boyce T, et al. Health Equity in England: The Marmot Review 10 Years On. London: Institute of Health Equity, 2020.

Marmot MG, Kogevinas M, Elston MA. Social/economic status and disease. Annu Rev Public Health 1987;8:111-35.

Marmot MG, Rose G, Shipley M, Hamilton PJ. Employment grade and coronary heart disease in British civil servants. J Epidemiol Community Health 1978;32:244-9.

Marmot MG, Shipley MJ, Rose G. Inequalities in death--specific explanations of a general pattern? Lancet 1984;1(8384):1003-6.

Marmot MG, Smith GD, Stansfeld S, et al. Health inequalities among British civil servants: the Whitehall II study. Lancet. 1991;337:1387-93.

Martens DS, Janssen BG, Bijnens EM, et al. Association of parental socioeconomic status and newborn telomere length. JAMA Netw Open 2020;3:e204057.

Martinson ML. Income inequality in health at all ages: a comparison of the United States and England. Am J Public Health 2012;102:2049-56.

Pickett KE, Wilkinson RG. Income inequality and health: a causal review. Soc Sci Med 2015;128:316-26.

Pool LR, Burgard SA, Needham BL, et al. Association of a negative wealth shock with all-cause mortality in middle-aged and older adults in the United States. JAMA 2018;319:1341-50.

Powell-Wiley TM, Gebreab SY, Claudel SE, et al. The relationship between neighborhood socioeconomic deprivation and telomere length. SSM Popul Health 2019;10:100517.

Roelfs DJ, Shor E, Davidson KW, Schwartz JE. Losing life and livelihood: a systematic review and meta-analysis of unemployment and all-cause mortality. Soc Sci Med 2011;72:840-54.

Sapolsky RM. The influence of social hierarchy on primate health. Science 2005;308:648–52.

Sapolsky RM. The health-wealth gap. Sci Am 2018;319(5):62-7.

Schencker L. Chicago's lifespan gap: Streeterville residents live to 90. Englewood residents die at 60. Study finds it's the largest divide in the U.S. Chicago Tribune, June 6, 2019.

Strandberg TE, Räikkönen K, Salomaa V, et al. Increased mortality despite successful multifactorial cardiovascular risk reduction in healthy men: 40-year follow-up of the Helsinki Businessmen Study Intervention Trial. J Nutr Health Aging 2018;22:885-91.

van den Heuvel WJ, Olaroiu M. How important are health care expenditures for life expectancy? A comparative, European analysis. J Am Med Dir Assoc 2017;18:276.e9-12.

Vineis P, Delpierre C, Castagné R, et al. Health inequalities: embodied evidence across biological layers. Soc Sci Med 2020;246:112781.

For life expectancies and London Underground tube stations, see https://tubecreature.com/#/livesontheline/current/same/*/*/FFTFTF/13/-0.1000/51.5200/ (accessed April 13, 2020).

22. Pressure Drop

ALLHAT Collaborative Research Group. Major outcomes in high-risk hypertensive patients randomized to angiotensin-converting enzyme inhibitor or calcium channel blocker vs diuretic: The Antihypertensive and Lipid-Lowering Treatment to Prevent Heart Attack Trial (ALLHAT). JAMA 2002;288:2981-97.

Appel LJ, Moore TJ, Obarzanek E, et al. A clinical trial of the effects of dietary patterns on blood pressure. DASH Collaborative Research Group. N Engl J Med 1997;336:1117-24.

Cohen IB. Stephen Hales. Sci Am 1976;234:98-107.

Dorans KS, Mills KT, Liu Y, He J. Trends in prevalence and control of hypertension according to the 2017 American College of Cardiology/American Heart Association (ACC/AHA) Guideline. J Am Heart Assoc 2018;7:e008888.

Evans H. Losing touch: the controversy over the introduction of blood pressure instruments into medicine. Technol Cult 1993;34:784-807.

Fisher JW. The diagnostic value of the sphygmomanometer in examinations for life insurance. JAMA 1914;63:1752-4.

Forette F, Seux ML, Staessen JA, et al. The prevention of dementia with antihypertensive treatment: new evidence from the Systolic Hypertension in Europe (Syst-Eur) study. Arch Intern Med 2002;162:2046-52.

Hales S. Statical Essays. London: William Innys and Richard Manby, 1733.

Klein AV, Kiat H. The mechanisms underlying fructose-induced hypertension: a review. J Hypertens 2015;33:912-20.

Moser M. Historical perspectives on the management of hypertension. J Clin Hypertens (Greenwich) 2006;8(8 Suppl 2):15-39.

Musini VM, Gueyffier F, Puil L, et al. Pharmacotherapy for hypertension in adults aged 18 to 59 years. Cochrane Database Syst Rev 2017;8(8): CD008276.

Musini VM, Tejani AM, Bassett K, et al. Pharmacotherapy for hypertension in adults 60 years or older. Cochrane Database Syst Rev 2019;6(6): CD000028.

SPRINT MIND Investigators for the SPRINT Research Group, Williamson JD, Pajewski NM, et al. Effect of intensive vs standard blood pressure control on probable dementia. JAMA 2019;321:553-561.

Unger T, Borghi C, Charchar F, et al. 2020 International Society of Hypertension global hypertension practice guidelines. J Hypertens 2020; 38:982-1004.

Whelton PK, Carey RM, Aronow WS, et al. 2017 ACC/AHA/AAPA/ABC/ACPM/AGS/APhA/ASH/ASPC/NMA/PCNA guideline for the prevention, detection, evaluation, and management of high blood pressure in adults. Circulation 2018;138:e484-e594.

23. The Weight

Abdelhamid AS, Brown TJ, Brainard JS, et al. Omega-3 fatty acids for the primary and secondary prevention of cardiovascular disease. Cochrane Database Syst Rev 2020;3(2):CD003177.

Althoff T, Sosič R, Hicks JL, et al. Large-scale physical activity data reveal worldwide activity inequality. Nature 2017;547:336-9.

Aune D, Sen A, Prasad M, et al. BMI and all cause mortality: systematic review and non-linear dose-response meta-analysis of 230 cohort studies with 3.74 million deaths among 30.3 million participants. BMJ 2016;353:i2156.

Bao Y, Han J, Hu FB, et al. Association of nut consumption with total and cause-specific mortality. N Engl J Med 2013;369:2001-11.

Bassett DR, Schneider PL, Huntington GE. Physical activity in an Old Order Amish community. Med Sci Sports Exerc 2004;36:79-85.

Bertoia ML, Mukamal KJ, Cahill LE, et al. Changes in intake of fruits and vegetables and weight change in United States men and women followed for up to 24 years. PLoS Med 2015;12(9):e1001878.

Carroll A. The Bad Food Bible. Boston: Houghton Mifflin Harcourt, 2017.

Cardoso L, Rodrigues D, Gomes L, Carrilho F. Short- and long-term mortality after bariatric surgery: systematic review and meta-analysis. Diabetes Obes Metab 2017;19:1223-32.

de Souza RJ, Mente A, Maroleanu A, et al. Intake of saturated and trans unsaturated fatty acids and risk of all cause mortality, cardiovascular disease, and type 2 diabetes: systematic review and meta-analysis of observational studies. BMJ 2015;351:h3978.

Dehghan M, Mente A, Zhang X, et al. Associations of fats and carbohydrate intake with cardiovascular disease and mortality in 18 countries from five continents (PURE): a prospective cohort study. Lancet 2017;390(10107):2050-62.

Delaney B, Walford L. The Longevity Diet: The Only Proven Way to Slow the Aging Process and Maintain Peak Vitality Through Caloric Restriction. Cambridge: Da Capo Press, 2010.

Fulwiler C, Brewer JA, Sinnott S, Loucks EB. Mindfulness-based interventions for weight loss and CVD risk management. Curr Cardiovasc Risk Rep 2015;9(10):46.

Guo J, Astrup A, Lovegrove JA, Gijsbers L, Givens DI, Soedamah-Muthu SS. Milk and dairy consumption and risk of cardiovascular diseases and all-cause mortality: dose-response meta-analysis of prospective cohort studies. Eur J Epidemiol 2017;32:269-87.

Hales CM, Carroll MD, Fryar CD, Ogden CL. Prevalence of obesity and severe obesity among adults: United States, 2017–2018. NCHS Data Brief, no 360. Hyattsville, MD: National Center for Health Statistics, 2020.

Hooper L, Martin N, Jimoh OF, et al. Reduction in saturated fat intake for cardiovascular disease. Cochrane Database Syst Rev 2020;5:CD011737.

Kokkinos P, Faselis C, Myers J, et al. Cardiorespiratory fitness and the paradoxical BMI-mortality risk association in male veterans. Mayo Clin Proc 2014;89:754-762.

Li ZH, Zhong WF, Liu S, et al. Associations of habitual fish oil supplementation with cardiovascular outcomes and all cause mortality. BMJ 2020;368:m456.

Linder CR. Adaptive evolution of seed oils in plants: accounting for the biogeographic distribution of saturated and unsaturated fatty acids in seed oils. Am Nat 2000;156:442-58.

Lowe DA, Wu N, Rohdin-Bibby L, et al. Effects of time-restricted eating on weight loss and other metabolic parameters in women and men with overweight and obesity: the TREAT randomized clinical trial. JAMA Intern Med 2020;180:1–9.

Jayedi A, Shab-Bidar S. Fish consumption and the risk of chronic disease: an umbrella review of meta-analyses of prospective cohort studies. Adv Nutr 2020;nmaa029.

Johnston BC, Kanters S, Bandayrel K, et al. Comparison of weight loss among named diet programs in overweight and obese adults: a meta-analysis. JAMA 2014;312:923-33.

Manheimer EW, van Zuuren EJ, Fedorowicz Z, Pijl H. Paleolithic nutrition for metabolic syndrome: systematic review and meta-analysis. Am J Clin Nutr 2015;102:922-32.

Mazidi M, Mikhailidis DP, Sattar N, et al. Association of types of dietary fats and all-cause and cause-specific mortality: prospective cohort study and meta-analysis of prospective studies with 1,164,029 participants. Clin Nutr 2020;S0261-5614(20)30146-1.

Mozaffarian D, Hao T, Rimm EB, et al. Changes in diet and lifestyle and long-term weight gain in women and men. N Engl J Med 2011;364:2392-2404.

Noguchi Y. My new diet is an app: weight loss goes digital. NPR, April 15, 2019.

O'Neill B, Raggi P. The ketogenic diet: pros and cons. Atherosclerosis 2020; 292:119-26.

Sacks FM, Bray GA, Carey VJ, et al. Comparison of weight-loss diets with different compositions of fat, protein, and carbohydrates. N Engl J Med 2009;360:859-73.

Schwingshackl L, Schwedhelm S, Hoffmann G, et al. Food groups and risk of all-cause mortality: a systematic review and meta-analysis of prospective studies. Am J Clin Nutr 2017;105:1462–73.

Sievert K, Hussain SM, Page MJ, et al. Effect of breakfast on weight and energy intake: systematic review and meta-analysis of randomised controlled trials. BMJ 2019;364:l42.

Smith JD, Hou T, Ludwig DS, et al. Changes in intake of protein foods, carbohydrate amount and quality, and long-term weight change: results from 3 prospective cohorts. Am J Clin Nutr 2015;101:1216-24.

Teicholz N. The Big Fat Surprise. New York: Simon and Schuster, 2014.

van Strien T. Causes of emotional eating and matched treatment of obesity. Curr Diab Rep 2018;18(6):35.

Villablanca PA, Alegria JR, Mookadam F, et al. Nonexercise activity thermogenesis in obesity management. Mayo Clin Proc 2015;90:509-19.

Wang DD, Hu FB. Dietary fat and risk of cardiovascular disease: recent controversies and advances. Annu Rev Nutr 2017;37:423-446.

24. Moral Fiber

Aune D, Sen A, Norat T, Riboli E. Dietary fibre intake and the risk of diverticular disease: a systematic review and meta-analysis of prospective studies. Eur J Nutr 2020;59:421-32.

Bozzetto L, Costabile G, Della Pepa G, et al. Dietary fibre as a unifying remedy for the whole spectrum of obesity-associated cardiovascular risk. Nutrients 2018;10:943.

Eakin E. The excrement experiment. The New Yorker, December 1, 2014.

Eiseman B, Silen W, Bascom GS, Kauvar AJ. Fecal enema as an adjunct in the treatment of pseudomembranous enterocolitis. Surgery 1958; 44:854-9.

Hills RD Jr, Pontefract BA, Mishcon HR, et al. Gut microbiome: profound implications for diet and disease. Nutrients 2019;11:1613.

Khanna S, Tosh PK. A clinician's primer on the role of the microbiome in human health and disease. Mayo Clin Proc 2014;89:107-114.

Khoruts A. Fecal microbiota transplantation-early steps on a long journey ahead. Gut Microbes 2017;8:199-204.

Liu L, Wang S, Liu J. Fiber consumption and all-cause, cardiovascular, and cancer mortalities: a systematic review and meta-analysis of cohort studies. Mol Nutr Food Res 2015;59:139-146.

Magne F, Gotteland M, Gauthier L, et al. The Firmicutes/Bacteroidetes ratio: a relevant marker of gut dysbiosis in obese patients?. Nutrients 2020;12:1474.

Nagpal R, Mainali R, Ahmadi S, et al. Gut microbiome and aging: Physiological and mechanistic insights. Nutr Healthy Aging 2018;4:267-285.

Santos-Marcos JA, Perez-Jimenez F, Camargo A. The role of diet and intestinal microbiota in the development of metabolic syndrome. J Nutr Biochem 2019;70:1-27.

Soliman GA. Dietary fiber, atherosclerosis, and cardiovascular disease. Nutrients 2019;11:1155.

Yang Y, Zhao LG, Wu QJ, et al. Association between dietary fiber and lower risk of all-cause mortality: a meta-analysis of cohort studies. Am J Epidemiol 2015;181:83-91.

25. Only the Good Die Old

Friedman HS, Martin LR. The Longevity Project. New York: Hudson Street Press, 2011.

Javaras KN, Williams M, Baskin-Sommers AR. Psychological interventions potentially useful for increasing conscientiousness. Personal Disord 2019;10:13-24.

Kern ML, Friedman HS. Do conscientious individuals live longer? A quantitative review. Health Psychol 2008;27:505-12.

Lawrence EM, Rogers RG, Wadsworth T. Happiness and longevity in the United States. Soc Sci Med 2015;145:115-9.

Liu B, Floud S, Pirie K, et al. Does happiness itself directly affect mortality? The prospective UK Million Women Study. Lancet 2016;387:874-81.

Steptoe A, Deaton A, Stone AA. Subjective wellbeing, health, and ageing. Lancet 2015;385:640-8.

Terracciano A, Löckenhoff CE, Zonderman AB, et al. Personality predictors of longevity: activity, emotional stability, and conscientiousness. Psychosom Med 2008;70:621-7.

Vaillant GE. Triumphs of Experience: The Men of the Harvard Grant Study. Cambridge, Harvard University Press, 2012:247-9.

26. Marriage Story

Chen R, Zhan Y, Pedersen N, et al. Marital status, telomere length and cardiovascular disease risk in a Swedish prospective cohort. Heart 2020; 106:267-72.

Choi H, Marks NF. Socioeconomic status, marital status continuity and change, marital conflict, and mortality. J Aging Health 2011;23:714-42.

Friedman HS, Martin LR. The Longevity Project. New York: Hudson Street Press, 2011.

Frisch M, Simonsen J. Marriage, cohabitation and mortality in Denmark: national cohort study of 6.5 million persons followed for up to three decades (1982-2011). Int J Epidemiol 2013;42:559-78.

Hatzenbuehler ML, O'Cleirigh C, Grasso C, et al. Effect of same-sex marriage laws on health care use and expenditures in sexual minority men: a quasi-natural experiment. Am J Public Health 2012;102:285-91.

Ikeda A, Iso H, Toyoshima H, et al. Marital status and mortality among Japanese men and women: the Japan Collaborative Cohort Study. BMC Public Health 2007;7:73.

Kaplan RM, Kronick RG. Marital status and longevity in the United States population. J Epidemiol Community Health 2006;60:760-5.

Martikainen P, Valkonen T. Mortality after the death of a spouse: rates and causes of death in a large Finnish cohort. Am J Public Health 1996;86: 1087-93.

Mata J, Frank R, Hertwig R. Higher body mass index, less exercise, but healthier eating in married adults: nine representative surveys across Europe. Soc Sci Med 2015;138:119-27.

Tucker JS, Friedman HS, Wingard DL, Schwartz JE. Marital history at midlife as a predictor of longevity: alternative explanations to the protective effect of marriage. Health Psychol 1996;15:94-101.

Tuller D. The health effects of legalizing same-sex marriage. Health Aff (Millwood) 2017;36:978-81.

Va P, Yang WS, Nechuta S, et al. Marital status and mortality among middle age and elderly men and women in urban Shanghai. PLoS One 2011; 6(11):e26600.

Wang Y, Jiao Y, Nie J, et al. Sex differences in the association between marital status and the risk of cardiovascular, cancer, and all-cause mortality: a systematic review and meta-analysis of 7,881,040 individuals. Glob Health Res Policy 2020;5:4.

Whisman MA, Robustelli BL, Sbarra DA. Marital disruption is associated with shorter salivary telomere length in a probability sample of older adults. Soc Sci Med 2016;157:60-7.

Wight RG, Leblanc AJ, Lee Badgett MV. Same-sex legal marriage and psychological well-being: findings from the California Health Interview Survey. Am J Public Health 2013;103:339-46.

27. Gotta Serve Somebody

Ajdacic-Gross V, Knöpfli D, Landolt K, et al. Death has a preference for birthdays-an analysis of death time series. Ann Epidemiol 2012;22:603-6.

Anderson ND, Damianakis T, Kröger E, et al. The benefits associated with volunteering among seniors: a critical review and recommendations for future research. Psychol Bull 2014;140:1505-33.

Chen Y, Kim ES, VanderWeele TJ. Religious-service attendance and subsequent health and well-being throughout adulthood: evidence from three prospective cohorts. Int J Epidemiol 2020;dyaa120.

Cohen R, Bavishi C, Rozanski A. Purpose in life and its relationship to all-cause mortality and cardiovascular events: a meta-analysis. Psychosom Med 2016;78:122-33.

Frankl VE. Man's Search for Meaning. Boston: Beacon Press, 2006.

Grimm R, Spring K, Dietz N. The Health Benefits of Volunteering: A Review of Recent Research. Washington, DC: Corporation for National and Community Service, Office of Research and Policy, 2007.

Inagaki TK, Bryne Haltom KE, Suzuki S, et al. The neurobiology of giving versus receiving support: the role of stress-related and social reward-related neural activity. Psychosom Med 2016;78:443-53.

Inagaki TK, Eisenberger NI. Giving support to others reduces sympathetic nervous system-related responses to stress. Psychophysiology 2016;53:427-435.

Kim ES, Whillans AV, Lee MT, et al. Volunteering and subsequent health and well-being in older adults. Am J Prev Med 2020;59:176-86.

McCullough ME, Hoyt WT, Larson DB, et al. Religious involvement and mortality: a meta-analytic review. Health Psychol 2000;19:211-222.

Okun MA, Yeung EW, Brown S. Volunteering by older adults and risk of mortality: a meta-analysis. Psychol Aging 2013;28:564-77.

Pytell T. The missing pieces of the puzzle: a reflection on the odd career of Viktor Frankl. J Contemp Hist 2000;35:281-306.

Sone T, Nakaya N, Ohmori K, et al. Sense of life worth living (ikigai) and mortality in Japan: Ohsaki Study. Psychosom Med 2008;70:709-15.

Whillans AV, Dunn EW, Sandstrom GM, et al. Is spending money on others good for your heart? Health Psychol 2016;35:574-583.

28. Java Jive

Astrup A, Toubro S, Cannon S, et al. Caffeine: a double-blind, placebo-controlled study of its thermogenic, metabolic, and cardiovascular effects in healthy volunteers. Am J Clin Nutr 1990;51:759-67.

Bonaccio M, Di Castelnuovo A, Costanzo S, et al. Chili pepper consumption and mortality in Italian adults. J Am Coll Cardiol 2019;74:3139-49.

Chopan M, Littenberg B. The association of hot red chili pepper consumption and mortality: a large population-based cohort study. PLoS One 2017;12:e0169876.

Chrysant SG. Coffee consumption and cardiovascular health. Am J Cardiol 2015;116:818-821.

Chung M, Zhao N, Wang D, et al. Dose-response relation between tea consumption and risk of cardiovascular disease and all-cause mortality. Adv Nutr 2020; nmaa010.

Clark KS, Coleman C, Shelton R, et al. Caffeine enhances activity thermogenesis and energy expenditure in rats. Clin Exp Pharmacol Physiol 2019;46:475-82.

Dulloo AG, Geissler CA, Horton T, et al. Normal caffeine consumption: influence on thermogenesis and daily energy expenditure in lean and postobese human volunteers. Am J Clin Nutr 1989;49:44-50.

Freedman ND, Park Y, Abnet CC, et al. Association of coffee drinking with total and cause-specific mortality. N Engl J Med 2012;366:1891-1904.

Harpaz E, Tamir S, Weinstein A, Weinstein Y. The effect of caffeine on energy balance. J Basic Clin Physiol Pharmacol 2017;28:1-10.

In praise of tea. Br Med J 1937;2(4016):529-30.

Kim Y, Je Y, Giovannucci E. Coffee consumption and all-cause and cause-specific mortality: a meta-analysis by potential modifiers. Eur J Epidemiol 2019;34:731-52.

Lee AH, Kabashneh S, Tsouvalas CP, et al. Proctocolitis from coffee enema. ACG Case Rep J 2020;7(1):e00292.

LeBlanc J, Jobin M, Côté J, Samson P, Labrie A. Enhanced metabolic response to caffeine in exercise-trained human subjects. J Appl Physiol 1985;59:832-7.

Loftfield E, Freedman ND, Dodd KW, et al. Coffee drinking is widespread in the United States, but usual intake varies by key demographic and lifestyle factors. J Nutr 2016;146:1762-8.

Pauli S. A Treatise on Tobacco, Tea, Coffee, and Chocolate. London: T. Osborne, 1746.

Poehlman ET, Després JP, Bessette H, et al. Influence of caffeine on the resting metabolic rate of exercise-trained and inactive subjects. Med Sci Sports Exerc 1985;17:689-94.

Poole R, Kennedy OJ, Roderick P, et al. Coffee consumption and health: umbrella review of meta-analyses of multiple health outcomes. BMJ 2017;359:j5024.

Schama S. Citizens: A Chronicle of the French Revolution. New York: Knopf, 1989.

Stuart C. A Proclamation for the Suppression of the Coffee-Houses. London: John Bill and Christopher Barker, 1675.

Tajik N, Tajik M, Mack I, Enck P. The potential effects of chlorogenic acid, the main phenolic components in coffee, on health: a comprehensive review of the literature. Eur J Nutr 2017;56:2215-44.

Tsujimoto T, Kajio H, Sugiyama T. Association between caffeine intake and all-cause and cause-specific mortality. Mayo Clin Proc 2017;92: 1190-1202.

Urgert R, Katan MB. The cholesterol-raising factor from coffee beans. Annu Rev Nutr 1997;17:305-24.

29. Brain Drain

Biazus-Sehn LF, Schuch FB, Firth J, Stigger FS. Effects of physical exercise on cognitive function of older adults with mild cognitive impairment: a systematic review and meta-analysis. Arch Gerontol Geriatr 2020;89:1040-8.

De la Rosa A, Olaso-Gonzalez G, Arc-Chagnaud C, et al. Physical exercise in the prevention and treatment of Alzheimer's disease. J Sport Health Sci 2020;9:394-404.

Erickson KI, Voss MW, Prakash RS, et al. Exercise training increases size of hippocampus and improves memory. Proc Natl Acad Sci USA 2011; 108:3017-22.

Fan L, Mao C, Hu X, et al. New insights into the pathogenesis of Alzheimer's disease. Front Neurol 2020;10:1312.

Farfel JM, Yu L, Boyle PA, et al. Alzheimer's disease frequency peaks in the tenth decade and is lower afterwards. Acta Neuropathol Commun 2019;7(1):104.

Gao S, Burney HN, Callahan CM, Purnell CE, Hendrie HC. Incidence of dementia and Alzheimer disease over time: a meta-analysis. J Am Geriatr Soc 2019;67:1361-9.

Gates NJ, Rutjes AW, Di Nisio M, et al. Computerised cognitive training for maintaining cognitive function in cognitively healthy people in midlife. Cochrane Database Syst Rev 2019;3(3):CD012278.

Gates NJ, Vernooij RW, Di Nisio M, et al. Computerised cognitive training for preventing dementia in people with mild cognitive impairment. Cochrane Database Syst Rev 2019;3(3):CD012279.

Graeber MB, Kösel S, Grasbon-Frodl E, et al. Histopathology and APOE genotype of the first Alzheimer disease patient, Auguste D. Neurogenetics 1998;1:223-8.

He Q, Chen X, Wu T, et al. Risk of dementia in long-term benzodiazepine users: evidence from a meta-analysis of observational studies. J Clin Neurol 2019;15:9-19.

Hughes TF, Chang CC, Vander Bilt J, Ganguli M. Engagement in reading and hobbies and risk of incident dementia: the MoVIES project. Am J Alzheimers Dis Other Demen 2010;25:432-8.

Liu PZ, Nusslock R. Exercise-mediated neurogenesis in the hippocampus via BDNF. Front Neurosci 2018;12:52.

Livingston G, Huntley J, Sommerlad A, et al. Dementia prevention, intervention, and care: 2020 report of the Lancet Commission. Lancet 2020;396:413-46.

Maurer K, Volk S, Gerbaldo H. Auguste D and Alzheimer's disease. Lancet 1997;349:1546-9.

Morris JC. Is Alzheimer's disease inevitable with age? J Clin Invest 1999; 104:1171-3.

Nedergaard M, Goldman SA. Glymphatic failure as a final common pathway to dementia. Science 2020;370:50-56.

Pillai JA, Hall CB, Dickson DW, et al. Association of crossword puzzle participation with memory decline in persons who develop dementia. J Int Neuropsychol Soc 2011;17:1006-13.

Ratey JJ, Hagerman E. Spark: The Revolutionary New Science of Exercise and the Brain. New York: Little, Brown and Company, 2008.

Saito T, Murata C, Saito M, et al. Influence of social relationship domains and their combinations on incident dementia: a prospective cohort study. J Epidemiol Community Health 2018;72:7-12.

Sommerlad A, Sabia S, Singh-Manoux A, et al. Association of social contact with dementia and cognition: 28-year follow-up of the Whitehall II cohort study. PLoS Med;16(8):e1002862.

Staff RT, Hogan MJ, Williams DS, Whalley LJ. Intellectual engagement and cognitive ability in later life (the "use it or lose it" conjecture): longitudinal, prospective study. BMJ 2018;363:k4925.

Steptoe A, Hamer M, Butcher L, et al. Educational attainment but not measures of current socioeconomic circumstances are associated with leukocyte telomere length in healthy older men and women. Brain Behav Immun 2011;25:1292-8.

Valenzuela MJ, Sachdev P. Brain reserve and dementia: a systematic review. Psychol Med 2006;36:441-54.

Verghese J, Lipton RB, Katz MJ, et al. Leisure activities and the risk of dementia in the elderly. N Engl J Med 2003;348:2508-16.

SPRINT MIND Investigators for the SPRINT Research Group, Williamson JD, Pajewski NM, Auchus AP, et al. Effect of intensive vs standard blood pressure control on probable dementia: a randomized clinical trial. JAMA 2019;321:553-61.

Wilson RS, Li Y, Aggarwal NT, et al. Education and the course of cognitive decline in Alzheimer disease. Neurology 2004;63:1198-202.

Yang HD, Kim DH, Lee SB, Young LD. History of Alzheimer's disease. Dement Neurocogn Disord 2016;15:115-21.

Yang K, Zhang Y, Saito E, et al. Association between educational level and total and cause-specific mortality: a pooled analysis of over 694 000 individuals in the Asia Cohort Consortium. BMJ Open 2019;9(8):e026225.

30. Running Up That Hill

Allard M, Lèbre V, Robine JM. Jeanne Calment: From Van Gogh's Time to Ours. New York: WH Freeman, 1998.

Arsenis NC, You T, Ogawa EF, et al. Physical activity and telomere length: impact of aging and potential mechanisms of action. Oncotarget 2017;8:45008-19.

Chen ZP, Stephens TJ, Murthy S, et al. Effect of exercise intensity on skeletal muscle AMPK signaling in humans. Diabetes 2003;52:2205-12.

Collins L. Was Jeanne Calment the oldest person who ever lived—or a fraud? New Yorker, February 10, 2020.

DiMenna FJ, Arad AD. Exercise as 'precision medicine' for insulin resistance and its progression to type 2 diabetes. BMC Sports Sci Med Rehabil 2018;10:21.

Domenech-Ximenos B, Sanz-de la Garza M, Prat-González S, et al. Prevalence and pattern of cardiovascular magnetic resonance late gadolinium enhancement in highly trained endurance athletes. J Cardiovasc Magn Reson 2020;22:62.

Gronek P, Wielinski D, Cyganski P, et al. A review of exercise as medicine in cardiovascular disease: pathology and mechanism. Aging Dis 2020; 11:327-340.

Jeune B, Robine J-M, Young R, et al. Jeanne Calment and her successors. Biographical notes on the longest living humans. In: Maier H, Gampe J, Jeune B, Robine J-M, Vaupel JW, editors. Supercentenarians. Berlin, Heidelberg: Springer; 2010. p. 285–323.

Lee IM, Shiroma EJ, Kamada M, et al. Association of step volume and intensity with all-cause mortality in older women. JAMA Intern Med 2019;179:1105–12.

McGee SL, Hargreaves M. Exercise adaptations: molecular mechanisms and potential targets for therapeutic benefit. Nat Rev Endocrinol 2020; 16:495-505.

Mishima RS, Verdicchio CV, Noubiap JJ, et al. Self-reported physical activity and atrial fibrillation risk: A systematic review and meta-analysis. Heart Rhythm 2020 Dec 19:S1547-5271(20)31165-6.

Naci H, Ioannidis JP. Comparative effectiveness of exercise and drug interventions on mortality outcomes: metaepidemiological study. Br J Sports Med 2015;49:1414-22.

O'Donovan G, Lee I, Hamer M, Stamatakis E. Association of "weekend war-
rior" and other leisure time physical activity patterns with risks for all-
cause, cardiovascular disease, and cancer mortality. JAMA Intern Med
2017;177:335–42.

O'Keefe JH, Franklin B, Lavie CJ. Exercising for health and longevity vs
peak performance: different regimens for different goals. Mayo Clin
Proc 2014;89:1171-5.

Pedisic Z, Shrestha N, Kovalchik S, et al. Is running associated with a
lower risk of all-cause, cardiovascular and cancer mortality, and is the
more better? A systematic review and meta-analysis. Br J Sports Med
2020;54:898-905.

Piercy KL, Troiano RP, Ballard RM, et al. The Physical Activity Guidelines
for Americans. JAMA 2018;320:2020-8.

Puterman E, Lin J, Blackburn E, O'Donovan A, et al. The power of exercise:
buffering the effect of chronic stress on telomere length. PLoS One
2010;5(5):e10837.

Radák Z, Apor P, Pucsok J, et al. Marathon running alters the DNA base ex-
cision repair in human skeletal muscle. Life Sci 2003;72:1627-33.

Rebelo-Marques A, De Sousa Lages A, Andrade R, et al. Aging hallmarks: the
benefits of physical exercise. Front Endocrinol (Lausanne) 2018;9:258.

Robin-Champigneul F. Jeanne Calment's unique 122-year life span: facts
and factors; longevity history in her genealogical tree. Rejuvenation
Res 2020;23:19-47.

Saint-Maurice PF, Troiano RP, Bassett DR, et al. Association of daily step
count and step intensity with mortality among US adults. JAMA
2020;323:1151–60.

Svedberg N, Sundström J, James S, et al. Long-term incidence of atrial fibrillation and stroke among cross-country skiers. Circulation 2019;140:
910-20.

US Department of Health and Human Services. Physical Activity Guidelines
for Americans, 2nd ed. Washington, DC: US Department of Health and
Human Services, 2018.

Wang Y, Nie J, Ferrari G, et al. Association of physical activity intensity with
mortality: a national cohort study of 403 681 US adults. JAMA Intern
Med 2020:e206331.

Zhao M, Veeranki SP, Magnussen CG, Xi B. Recommended physical activity
and all cause and cause specific mortality in US adults: prospective cohort study. BMJ 2020;370:m2031.

31. State of Nature

Basu R, Pearson D, Malig B, et al. The effect of high ambient temperature on emergency room visits. Epidemiology 2012;23:813-820.

Beyer KM, Kaltenbach A, Szabo A, et al. Exposure to neighborhood green space and mental health: evidence from the survey of the health of Wisconsin. Int J Environ Res Public Health 2014;11:3453-72.

Branas CC, South E, Kondo MC, et al. Citywide cluster randomized trial to restore blighted vacant land and its effects on violence, crime, and fear. Proc Natl Acad Sci USA 2018;115:2946-51.

Brown H, Proust K, Newell B, et al. Cool communities: urban density, trees, and health. Int J Environ Res Public Health 2018;15(7):1547.

Donovan GH, Butry DT, Michael YL, et al. The relationship between trees and human health: evidence from the spread of the emerald ash borer. Am J Prev Med 2013;44:139–45.

Gascon M, Triguero-Mas M, Martínez D, et al. Residential green spaces and mortality: a systematic review. Environ Int 2016;86:60-7.

Helbich M, de Beurs D, Kwan MP, et al. Natural environments and suicide mortality in the Netherlands: a cross-sectional, ecological study. Lancet Planet Health 2018;2:e134-39.

Kardan O, Gozdyra P, Misic B, et al. Neighborhood greenspace and health in a large urban center. Sci Rep 2015;5:11610.

Kondo MC, Jacoby SF, South EC. Does spending time outdoors reduce stress? A review of real-time stress response to outdoor environments. Health Place 2018;51:136-50.

Maas J, van Dillen SME, Verheij RA, Groenewegen PP. Social contacts as a possible mechanism behind the relation between green space and health. Health Place 2009;15:586-95.

Mao GX, Cao YB, Lan XG, et al. Therapeutic effect of forest bathing on human hypertension in the elderly. J Cardiol 2012;60:495-502.

McMorris O, Villeneuve PJ, Su J, Jerrett M. Urban greenness and physical activity in a national survey of Canadians. Environ Res 2015;137:94-100.

Nowak DJ, Hirabayashi S, Bodine A, Greenfield E. Tree and forest effects on air quality and human health in the United States. Environ Pollut 2014;193:119–29.

Park MY, Chai CG, Lee HK, et al. The effects of natural daylight on length of hospital stay. Environ Health Insights 2018;12:1178630218812817.

Taylor MS, Wheeler BW, White MP, et al. Urban street tree density and antidepressant prescription rates: a cross-sectional study in London, UK. Landsc Urban Plan 2015;136:174-9.

Vant-Hull B, Karimi M, Sossa A, et al. Fine structure in Manhattan's daytime urban heat island. J Urban Environ Eng 2014;8:59-74.

Vienneau D, de Hoogh K, Faeh D, et al. More than clean air and tranquillity: residential green is independently associated with decreasing mortality. Environ Int 2017;108:176-84.

Villeneuve PJ, Jerrett M, Su JG, et al. A cohort study relating urban green space with mortality in Ontario, Canada. Environ Res 2012;115:51-8.

32. Hit Me With Your Best Shot

Anderson ML, Dobkin C, Gorry D. The effect of influenza vaccination for the elderly on hospitalization and mortality. Ann Intern Med 2020;172:445-52.

Arriola C, Garg S, Anderson EJ, et al. Influenza vaccination modifies disease severity among community-dwelling adults hospitalized with influenza. Clin Infect Dis 2017;65:1289-1297.

Baden LR, El Sahly HM, Essink B, et al; COVE Study Group. Efficacy and safety of the mRNA-1273 SARS-CoV-2 vaccine. N Engl J Med 2021;384:403-16.

Baldo V, Cocchio S, Gallo T, et al. Pneumococcal conjugated vaccine reduces the high mortality for community-acquired pneumonia in the elderly. PLoS One 2016;11:e0166637.

Cheng Y, Cao X, Cao Z, et al. Effects of influenza vaccination on the risk of cardiovascular and respiratory diseases and all-cause mortality. Ageing Res Rev 2020;62:101124.

Davidson JA, Banerjee A, Douglas I, et al. Primary prevention of acute cardiovascular events by influenza vaccination: an observational study. Eur Heart J. 2022 Dec 20:ehac737.

Demicheli V, Jefferson T, Di Pietrantonj C, et al. Vaccines for preventing influenza in the elderly. Cochrane Database Syst Rev 2018;2(2):CD004876.

Demicheli V, Jefferson T, Ferroni E, et al. Vaccines for preventing influenza in healthy adults. Cochrane Database Syst Rev 2018;2(2):CD001269.

DiazGranados CA, Dunning AJ, Kimmel M, et al. Efficacy of high-dose versus standard-dose influenza vaccine in older adults. N Engl J Med 2014;371:635-45.

Essink B, Sabharwal C, Cannon K, et al. Pivotal phase 3 randomized clinical trial of the safety, tolerability, and immunogenicity of 20-valent pneumococcal conjugate vaccine in adults aged ≥18 years. Clin Infect Dis 2022;75:390-8.

Fireman B, Lee J, Lewis N, et al. Influenza vaccination and mortality: differentiating vaccine effects from bias. Am J Epidemiol 2009;170:650-6.

Grant WB, Bhattoa HP, Boucher BJ. Seasonal variations of U.S. mortality rates: Roles of solar ultraviolet-B doses, vitamin D, gene expression, and infections. J Steroid Biochem Mol Biol 2017;173:5-12.

Huss A, Scott P, Stuck AE, et al. Efficacy of pneumococcal vaccination in adults: a meta-analysis. CMAJ 2009;180:48-58.

Kwong JC, Schwartz KL, Campitelli MA, et al. Acute myocardial infarction after laboratory-confirmed influenza infection. N Engl J Med 2018;378:345-53.

Lai FTT, Chan EWW, Huang L, et al. Prognosis of myocarditis developing after mRNA COVID-19 vaccination compared with viral myocarditis. J Am Coll Cardiol 2022;80:2255-65.

Marra F, Zhang A, Gillman E, et al. The protective effect of pneumococcal vaccination on cardiovascular disease in adults: a systematic review and meta-analysis. Int J Infect Dis 2020;99:204-13.

Marti-Soler H, Gonseth S, Gubelmann C, et al. Seasonal variation of overall and cardiovascular mortality: a study in 19 countries from different geographic locations. PLoS One 2014;9(11):e113500.

Massoud GP, Hazimeh DH, Amin G, et al. Risk of thromboembolic events in non-hospitalized COVID-19 patients: A systematic review. Eur J Pharmacol 2023 Feb 15;941:175501.

Moberley S, Holden J, Tatham DP, Andrews RM. Vaccines for preventing pneumococcal infection in adults. Cochrane Database Syst Rev 2013;2013(1):CD000422.

Nichol KL, Nordin JD, Nelson DB, Mullooly JP, Hak E. Effectiveness of influenza vaccine in the community-dwelling elderly. N Engl J Med 2007; 357:1373-81.

Nishiura H. Case fatality ratio of pandemic influenza. Lancet Infect Dis 2010;10:443-444.

Ohland J, Warren-Gash C, Blackburn R, et al. Acute myocardial infarctions and stroke triggered by laboratory-confirmed respiratory infections in Denmark, 2010 to 2016. Euro Surveill 2020;25(17):1900199.

Pálinkás A, Sándor J. Effectiveness of COVID-19 vaccination in preventing all-cause mortality among adults during the third wave of the epidemic in Hungary: nationwide retrospective cohort study. Vaccines (Basel) 2022;10:1009.

Pastor-Barriuso R, Pérez-Gómez B, Hernán MA, et al. Infection fatality risk for SARS-CoV-2 in community dwelling population of Spain: nationwide seroepidemiological study. BMJ 2020;371:m4509ht.

Patone M, Mei XW, Handunnetthi L, et al. Risk of myocarditis after sequential doses of COVID-19 vaccine and SARS-CoV-2 infection by age and sex. Circulation 2022;146:743-54.

Polack FP, Thomas SJ, Kitchin N, et al. C4591001 Clinical Trial Group. Safety and efficacy of the BNT162b2 mRNA Covid-19 vaccine. N Engl J Med 2020;383:2603-15.

Pop-Vicas A, Rahman M, Gozalo PL, et al. Estimating the effect of influenza vaccination on nursing home residents' morbidity and mortality. J Am Geriatr Soc 2015;63:1798-1804.

Reichert TA, Sugaya N, Fedson DS, et al. The Japanese experience with vaccinating schoolchildren against influenza. N Engl J Med 2001;344:889-96.

Tu W, Zhang P, Roberts A, et al. SARS-CoV-2 infection, hospitalization, and death in vaccinated and infected individuals by age groups in Indiana, 2021-2022. Am J Public Health 2023;113:96-104.

33. Screen Time

Arbyn M, Xu L, Simoens C, Martin-Hirsch PP. Prophylactic vaccination against human papillomaviruses to prevent cervical cancer and its precursors. Cochrane Database Syst Rev 2018;5(5):CD009069.

Borsky A, Zhan C, Miller T, et al. Few Americans receive all high-priority, appropriate clinical preventive services. Health Aff (Millwood) 2018;37:925-8.

Bretthauer M, Løberg M, Wieszczy P, et al.; NordICC Study Group. Effect of colonoscopy screening on risks of colorectal cancer and related death. N Engl J Med 2022;387:1547-56.

Chou R, Dana T, Blazina I, et al. Statins for prevention of cardiovascular disease in adults: evidence report and systematic review for the US Preventive Services Task Force. JAMA 2016;316:2008-24.

Curry SJ, Krist AH, Owens DK, et al. Screening for cervical cancer: US Preventive Services Task Force Recommendation Statement. JAMA 2018;320:674-86.

Darby SC, Ewertz M, McGale P, et al. Risk of ischemic heart disease in women after radiotherapy for breast cancer. N Engl J Med 2013;368:987-98.

de Bono JS, Guo C, Gurel B, et al. Prostate carcinogenesis: inflammatory storms. Nat Rev Cancer 2020;20:455-469.

de Koning HJ, van der Aalst CM, de Jong PA, et al. Reduced lung-cancer mortality with volume CT screening in a randomized trial. N Engl J Med 2020;382:503-513.

Ebell MH, Bentivegna M, Hulme C. Cancer-specific mortality, all-cause mortality, and overdiagnosis in lung cancer screening trials: a meta-analysis. Ann Fam Med 2020;18:545-52.

Fang F, Keating NL, Mucci LA, et al. Immediate risk of suicide and cardiovascular death after a prostate cancer diagnosis. J Natl Cancer Inst 2010;102:307-14.

Gelbenegger G, Postula M, Pecen L, et al. Aspirin for primary prevention of cardiovascular disease: a meta-analysis with a particular focus on subgroups. BMC Med 2019;17:198.

Gøtzsche PC, Jørgensen KJ. Screening for breast cancer with mammography. Cochrane Database Syst Rev 2013 Jun 4;2013(6):CD001877.

Huang KL, Wang SY, Lu WC, et al. Effects of low-dose computed tomography on lung cancer screening: a systematic review, meta-analysis, and trial sequential analysis. BMC Pulm Med 2019;19(1):126.

Ilic D, Djulbegovic M, Jung JH, et al. Prostate cancer screening with prostate-specific antigen (PSA) test: a systematic review and meta-analysis. BMJ 2018;362:k3519.

Jahn JL, Giovannucci EL, Stampfer MJ. The high prevalence of undiagnosed prostate cancer at autopsy: implications for epidemiology and treatment of prostate cancer in the prostate-specific antigen-era. Int J Cancer 2015;137:2795-802.

Lee JA, Chang Y, Kim Y, et al. Colonoscopic screening and risk of all-cause and colorectal cancer mortality in young and older individuals. Cancer Res Treat. 2022 Sep 20, epub ahead of print.

Ko MJ, Jo AJ, Kim YJ, et al. Time- and dose-dependent association of statin use with risk of clinically relevant new-onset diabetes mellitus in primary prevention: a nationwide observational cohort study. J Am Heart Assoc 2019;8(8):e011320.

Lin JS, Piper MA, Perdue LA, et al. Screening for colorectal cancer: updated evidence report and systematic review for the US Preventive Services Task Force. JAMA 2016;315:2576-94.

McNeil JJ, Gibbs P, Orchard SG, et al.; ASPREE Investigator Group. Effect of aspirin on cancer incidence and mortality in older adults. J Natl Cancer Inst 2020 Aug 11:djaa114.

McNeil JJ, Nelson MR, Woods RL, et al; ASPREE Investigator Group. Effect of aspirin on all-cause mortality in the healthy elderly. N Engl J Med 2018;379:1519-28.

Nelson HD, Fu R, Cantor A, et al. Effectiveness of breast cancer screening: systematic review and meta-analysis to update the 2009 U.S. Preventive Services Task Force Recommendation. Ann Intern Med 2016;164:244-55.

Nishihara R, Wu K, Lochhead P, et al. Long-term colorectal-cancer incidence and mortality after lower endoscopy. N Engl J Med 2013;369:1095-1105.

Peirson L, Fitzpatrick-Lewis D, Ciliska D, Warren R. Screening for cervical cancer: a systematic review and meta-analysis. Syst Rev 2013;2:35.

Prasad V, Lenzer J, Newman DH. Why cancer screening has never been shown to "save lives"--and what we can do about it. BMJ 2016;352:h6080.

Sankaranarayanan R, Nene BM, Shastri SS, et al. HPV screening for cervical cancer in rural India. N Engl J Med 2009;360:1385-94.

Siu AL; U.S. Preventive Services Task Force. Screening for breast cancer: U.S. Preventive Services Task Force Recommendation Statement. Ann Intern Med 2016;164:279-96.

Swartz AW, Eberth JM, Josey MJ, Strayer SM. Reanalysis of all-cause mortality in the US Preventive Services Task Force 2016 Evidence Report on Colorectal Cancer Screening. Ann Intern Med 2017;167:602-3.

Taylor F, Huffman MD, Macedo AF, et al. Statins for the primary prevention of cardiovascular disease. Cochrane Database Syst Rev 2013;2013(1): CD004816.

US Preventive Services Task Force. Screening for HIV infection: US Preventive Services Task Force Recommendation Statement. JAMA 2019; 321:2326–36.

Yaffe MJ, Mainprize JG. The value of all-cause mortality as a metric for assessing breast cancer screening. J Natl Cancer Inst 2020;112:989-93.

34. The Frailty of Our Powers

2019 American Geriatrics Society Beers Criteria® Update Expert Panel. American Geriatrics Society 2019 Updated AGS Beers Criteria® for Potentially Inappropriate Medication Use in Older Adults. J Am Geriatr Soc 2019;67:674-94.

Bjelakovic G, Gluud LL, Nikolova D, et al. Vitamin D supplementation for prevention of mortality in adults. Cochrane Database Syst Rev 2014 Jan 10;(1):CD007470.

Boettger SF, Angersbach B, Klimek CN, et al. Prevalence and predictors of vitamin D deficiency in frail older hospitalized patients. BMC Geriatr 2018;18:219.

Bolland MJ, Grey AB, Gamble GD, Reid IR. Effect of osteoporosis treatment on mortality: a meta-analysis. J Clin Endocrinol Metab 2010;95:1174-81.

Bray NW, Smart RR, Jakobi JM, Jones GR. Exercise prescription to reverse frailty. Appl Physiol Nutr Metab 2016;41:1112-6.

Cameron ID, Dyer SM, Panagoda CE, et al. Interventions for preventing falls in older people in care facilities and hospitals. Cochrane Database Syst Rev 2018 Sep 7;9:CD005465.

Gaksch M, Jorde R, Grimnes G, et al. Vitamin D and mortality: Individual participant data meta-analysis of standardized 25-hydroxyvitamin D in 26916 individuals from a European consortium. PLoS One 2017;12(2):e0170791.

Hauger AV, Bergland A, Holvik K, et al. Osteoporosis and osteopenia in the distal forearm predict all-cause mortality independent of grip strength. Osteoporos Int 2018;29:2447-56.

McLaughlin EC, El-Kotob R, Chaput JP, et al. Balance and functional training and health in adults: an overview of systematic reviews. Appl Physiol Nutr Metab 2020;45:S180-S196.

Tricco AC, Thomas SM, Veroniki AA, et al. Comparisons of interventions for preventing falls in older adults: a systematic review and meta-analysis. JAMA 2017;318:1687-99.

US Preventive Services Task Force. Screening for osteoporosis to prevent fractures: US Preventive Services Task Force Recommendation Statement. JAMA 2018;319:2521–31.

Wu L, Lin H, Hu Y, et al. The major causes and risk factors of total and cause-specific mortality during 5.4-year follow-up: the Shanghai Changfeng Study. Eur J Epidemiol 2019;34:939-49.

Xie Y, Bowe B, Yan Y, et al. Estimates of all-cause mortality and cause-specific mortality associated with proton pump inhibitors among US veterans: cohort study. BMJ 2019;365:l1580.

35. Enormous Changes at the Last Minute

Abad M, Mosteiro L, Pantoja C, et al. Reprogramming in vivo produces teratomas and iPS cells with totipotency features. Nature 2013;502:340-5.

Apolzan JW, Venditti EM, Edelstein SL, et al. Long-term weight loss with metformin or lifestyle intervention in the Diabetes Prevention Program Outcomes Study. Ann Intern Med 2019;170:682-90.

Bailey C, Day C. Metformin: its botanical background. Pract Diab Int 2004;21:115-7.

Bailey CJ. Metformin: historical overview. Diabetologia 2017;60:1566-76.

Barzilai N, Crandall JP, Kritchevsky SB, Espeland MA. Metformin as a tool to target aging. Cell Metab 2016;23:1060-5.

Bitto A, Ito TK, Pineda VV, LeTexier NJ, et al. Transient rapamycin treatment can increase lifespan and healthspan in middle-aged mice. Elife. 2016 Aug 23;5:e16351.

Campbell JM, Bellman SM, Stephenson MD, Lisy K. Metformin reduces all-cause mortality and diseases of ageing independent of its effect on diabetes control: A systematic review and meta-analysis. Ageing Res Rev 2017;40:31-44.

Christenson J, Whitby SJ, Mellor D, et al. The effects of resveratrol supplementation in overweight and obese humans: a systematic review of randomized trials. Metab Syndr Relat Disord 2016;14:323-33.

Conboy MJ, Conboy IM, Rando TA. Heterochronic parabiosis: historical perspective and methodological considerations for studies of aging and longevity. Aging Cell 2013;12:525-30.

Domecq JP, Prutsky G, Leppin A, et al. Drugs commonly associated with weight change: a systematic review and meta-analysis. J Clin Endocrinol Metab 2015;100:363-70.

Dudley HW, Rosenheim O, Starling WW. The constitution and synthesis of spermidine, a newly discovered base isolated from animal tissues. Biochem J 1927;21:97-103.

Dumas SN, Lamming DW. Next generation strategies for geroprotection via mTORC1 inhibition. J Gerontol A Biol Sci Med Sci 2020;75:14-23.

Eisenberg T, Abdellatif M, Schroeder S, et al. Cardioprotection and lifespan extension by the natural polyamine spermidine. Nat Med 2016;22:1428-38.

Fransquet PD, Wrigglesworth J, Woods RL, et al. The epigenetic clock as a predictor of disease and mortality risk: a systematic review and meta-analysis. Clin Epigenetics 2019;11:62.

Garratt M, Bower B, Garcia GG, Miller RA. Sex differences in lifespan extension with acarbose and 17-α estradiol: gonadal hormones underlie male-specific improvements in glucose tolerance and mTORC2 signaling. Aging Cell 2017;16:1256-66.

Glossmann HH, Lutz O. Metformin and aging: a review. Gerontology 2019; 65:581–90.

Gnesin F, Thuesen ACB, Kähler LKA, et al. Metformin monotherapy for adults with type 2 diabetes mellitus. Cochrane Database Syst Rev 2020;6(6):CD012906.

Gonzalez-Armenta JL, Li N, Lee RL, et al. Heterochronic parabiosis: old blood induces changes in mitochondrial structure and function of young mice. J Gerontol A Biol Sci Med Sci 2020 Dec 30:glaa299.

Greenberg MVC, Bourc'his D. The diverse roles of DNA methylation in mammalian development and disease. Nat Rev Mol Cell Biol 2019;20:590-607.

Halloran J, Hussong SA, Burbank R, et al. Chronic inhibition of mammalian target of rapamycin by rapamycin modulates cognitive and non-cognitive components of behavior throughout lifespan in mice. Neuroscience 2012;223:102-13.

Harrison DE, Strong R, Alavez S, et al. Acarbose improves health and lifespan in aging HET3 mice. Aging Cell 2019;18(2):e12898.

Hickson LJ, Langhi Prata LGP, Bobart SA, et al. Senolytics decrease senescent cells in humans: preliminary report from a clinical trial of dasatinib plus quercetin in individuals with diabetic kidney disease. EBioMedicine 2019;47:446-56.

Holman RR, Coleman RL, Chan JCN, et al. Effects of acarbose on cardiovascular and diabetes outcomes in patients with coronary heart disease and impaired glucose tolerance (ACE): a randomised, double-blind, placebo-controlled trial. Lancet Diabetes Endocrinol 2017;5:877-86.

Jeyaraman MM, Al-Yousif NSH, Singh Mann A, et al. Resveratrol for adults with type 2 diabetes mellitus. Cochrane Database Syst Rev 2020 Jan 17;1(1):CD011919.

Kahan BD. Discoverer of the treasure from a barren island: Suren Sehgal. Transplantation 2003;76:623-4.

Kane AE, Sinclair DA. Epigenetic changes during aging and their reprogramming potential. Crit Rev Biochem Mol Biol 2019;54:61-83.

Kang JS, Yang YR. Circulating plasma factors involved in rejuvenation. Aging (Albany NY) 2020;12:23394-408.

Kiechl S, Pechlaner R, Willeit P, et al. Higher spermidine intake is linked to lower mortality: a prospective population-based study. Am J Clin Nutr 2018;108:371-80.

Kulkarni AS, Gubbi S, Barzilai N. Benefits of metformin in attenuating the hallmarks of aging. Cell Metab 2020;32:15-30.

Liu H, Bravata DM, Olkin I, et al. Systematic review: the safety and efficacy of growth hormone in the healthy elderly. Ann Intern Med 2007;14:104-15.

Longo VD, Antebi A, Bartke A, et al. Interventions to slow aging in humans: are we ready? Aging Cell 2015;14:497-510.

Lunsford WR, McCay CM, Lupien PJ, et al. Parabiosis as a method for studying factors which affect aging in rats. Gerontologia 1963;7:1-8.

Madeo F, Hofer SJ, Pendl T, et al. Nutritional aspects of spermidine. Annu Rev Nutr 2020;40:135-59.

Moelands SV, Lucassen PL, Akkermans RP, et al. Alpha-glucosidase inhibitors for prevention or delay of type 2 diabetes mellitus and its associated complications in people at increased risk of developing type 2 diabetes mellitus. Cochrane Database Syst Rev 2018;12(12):CD005061.

Kulkarni AS, Gubbi S, Barzilai N. Benefits of metformin in attenuating the hallmarks of aging. Cell Metab 2020;32:15-30.

Pallauf K, Günther I, Kühn G, et al. The potential of resveratrol to act as a caloric restriction mimetic appears to be limited: insights from studies in mice. Adv Nutr 2020 Dec 3:nmaa148.

Partridge L, Fuentealba M, Kennedy BK. The quest to slow ageing through drug discovery. Nat Rev Drug Discov 2020;19:513-32.

Rasekh HR, Nazari P, Kamli-Nejad M, Hosseinzadeh L. Acute and subchronic oral toxicity of Galega officinalis in rats. J Ethnopharmacol 2008;116:21-6.

Ros M, Carrascosa JM. Current nutritional and pharmacological anti-aging interventions. Biochim Biophys Acta Mol Basis Dis 2019:165612.

Rosenheim O. The isolation of spermine phosphate from semen and testis. Biochem J 1924;18:1253-62.

Santiago-Fernández O, Osorio FG, Quesada V, et al. Development of a CRISPR/Cas9-based therapy for Hutchinson-Gilford progeria syndrome. Nat Med 2019;25:423-426.

Schreiber KH, Arriola Apelo SI, Yu D, et al. A novel rapamycin analog is highly selective for mTORC1 in vivo. Nat Commun 2019;10:3194.

Schwarz C, Benson GS, Horn N, et al. Effects of Spermidine Supplementation on Cognition and Biomarkers in Older Adults With Subjective Cognitive Decline: A Randomized Clinical Trial. JAMA Netw Open 2022;5(5):e2213875.

Triana-Martínez, F., Picallos-Rabina, P., Da Silva-Álvarez, S. et al. Identification and characterization of cardiac glycosides as senolytic compounds. Nat Commun 2019;10:4731.

Villeda SA, Plambeck KE, Middeldorp J, et al. Young blood reverses age-related impairments in cognitive function and synaptic plasticity in mice. Nat Med 2014;20:659-63.

Wilkinson HN, Hardman MJ. Senescence in wound repair: emerging strategies to target chronic healing wounds. Front Cell Dev Biol 2020;8:773.

Xu M, Pirtskhalava T, Farr JN, et al. Senolytics improve physical function and increase lifespan in old age. Nat Med 2018;24:1246-56.

Yang JH, Hayano M, Griffin PT, et al. Loss of epigenetic information as a cause of mammalian aging. Cell 2023 Jan 19;186(2):305-326.e27.

Yoo YJ, Kim H, Park SR, Yoon YJ. An overview of rapamycin: from discovery to future perspectives. J Ind Microbiol Biotechnol 2017;44:537-53

Zhu M, Meng P, Ling X, Zhou L. Advancements in therapeutic drugs targeting of senescence. Ther Adv Chronic Dis 2020;11:2040622320964125.

36. Last Things

Kavalieratos D, Corbelli J, Zhang D, et al. Association between palliative care and patient and caregiver outcomes: a systematic review and meta-analysis. JAMA 2016;316:2104-14.

Lum HD, Sudore RL, Bekelman DB. Advance care planning in the elderly. Med Clin North Am 2015;99:391-403.

Periyakoil VS, Neri E, Fong A, Kraemer H. Do unto others: doctors' personal end-of-life resuscitation preferences and their attitudes toward advance directives. PLoS One 2014;9(5):e98246.

Silveira MJ, Kim SY, Langa KM. Advance directives and outcomes of surrogate decision making before death. N Engl J Med 2010;362:1211-8.

Temel JS, Greer JA, Muzikansky A, et al. Early palliative care for patients with metastatic non-small-cell lung cancer. N Engl J Med 2010;363:733-42.

Yadav KN, Gabler NB, Cooney E, et al. Approximately one in three US adults completes any type of advance directive for end-of-life care. Health Aff (Millwood) 2017;36:1244-51.

Index

Note: **Bold** *page numbers indicate where a term is discussed as the main topic of a chapter.*

cortisol, 122, 126, 158, 184
cosmic rays, 9–11
COVID-19, 125, 190–91
Crohn's disease, 41, 148
Cutler, David, 120–22, 123
cyanobacteria, 27–28
cynical hostility, 68
cystic fibrosis, 32

Dachau, 162, 163
dasatinib, 212
dementia, *171–76*
    Alzheimer's disease, 33, 34, 73,
        169, 171–73
    amyotrophic lateral sclerosis
        (ALS) (Lou Gehrig's
        disease), 34, 52
    and anticholinergic drugs, 205
    and exercise, 179
    and high blood pressure, 136
    Lewy body dementia, 33
    and metformin, 211
    Parkinson's disease, 33, 34, 73,
        169
    and protein misfolding, 33–34
depression
    and alcohol, 102, 117
    and cynical hostility, 68
    and emotional eating, 145
    and exercise, 178
    and green space, 184, 185
    and loneliness/social isolation,
        115
    and poor appetite, 203
    and purpose in life, 161, 164
    and side effects of dietary
        supplements, 80
    and suicide, 103, 104, 105, 135
Desmoulins, Camille, 167–68
Deter, Auguste, 171–72, 176

diabetes
    and dementia, 175–76
    effects of longevity drugs, 210,
        211, 212, 213, 215
    and loneliness, 115
    nutritional factors, 63, 84, 92,
        99, 101, 142, 149, 169
    and physical activity, 109, 179
    and protein misfolding, 34
    and smoke/smoking, 72, 73
    and statin drugs, 193
    and stress hormones, 158
    treated with goat's rue, 210
    type 1, 144
    type 2, 17, 34, 63, 84, 92, 99,
        101, 142, 169, 179, 193
diet. See calorie restriction;
    nutrition
dietary supplements, 77–80
digoxin, 213
dinosaurs, 8, 12, 20
diverticulitis, 65, 148
DNA
    cancer caused by damage to,
        5–11, 29
    copied during cell division,
        2–3, 20
    damage from air pollution, 74
    damage from free radicals,
        29–30, 72, 109
    damage from stress, 126
    and evolution of reproduction,
        20–22
    methylation of, 216–17
    and premature aging diseases,
        2–4
    repair of, 8–9, 25, 35, 50, 53,
        179, 211, 215–17
    and telomeres, 3, 16–18, 126,
        159, 173, 179, 211

testosterone, 39–40, 117, 198
tetanus, 208
thyroid, 60
tissue culture, 14–16
tobacco. *See* smoke/smoking
Tolvajärvi, battle of, 61–62
tortoises, 16, 21–22
trans fats, 84, 142
trees, *183–86*
tuberculosis, 89, 126
tumors, 6–8, 22, 24–25, 79, 198,
    217. *See also* cancer
tumor suppressor genes, 8–9
turmeric, 77, 78, 80

ultraprocessed foods, 79, *81–87*,
    90–93, 94, 125, 136, 145, 148. *See
    also* meat
ultraviolet radiation, 11
United Kingdom, 78, 82, 107–8,
    111, 119–20, 122, 168, 176
United States
    air pollution, 73–75
    alcohol consumption, 98
    cancer statistics, 63, 194, 195,
        198
    cigarette industry, 71–72
    Cold War, 89
    diet, 44, 58, 64, 81, 84, 91,
        93–94, 141, 143, 145, 167
    dietary supplement industry,
        30, 77–78
    diet industry, 143–44
    end-of-life care, 222
    gun ownership, 104
    happiness, 152–53
    health insurance, 159
    income inequality and life
        expectancy, 120–27
    obesity, 145

sedentary lifestyle, 108, 145
suicide and murder rates, 40,
    103–4
urban green space, 183–85
vaccination, 188, 189

vaccinations, *187–91*
Vilcabamba, 114
vision, 78, 81, 117, 203, 217
vitamin D, 202–3
volunteering, 69, 118, 164
Vonnegut, Kurt, 31, 201

Walford, Lisa, 139
Walford, Roy, 43, 44–45, 46–47, 49,
    51, 52, 139
wealth, 25, 95, *119–30*, 152, 158,
    173, 178, 185
weight, *139–46*
    and blood pressure, 135, 136
    body mass index (BMI), 52,
        139–41, 144, 146, 178
    and caffeine, 169
    and dementia risk, 175
    and exercise, 179
    and nutrition, 52, 83–84, 85,
        92, 93, 141–46, 148–49
    and wealth/socioeconomic
        status, 120, 121, 125
    weight loss as effect of
        longevity drugs, 211, 213
    weight loss due to frailty, 201,
        203
Werner syndrome, 3, 17
whales, 21–22, 25
White, Paul Dudley, 134
Whitehall, 119–20, 122
whole foods, 114, 136, 144–45, 158,
    190, 207
wine, 101–2, 215

women. *See* men/women
  differences
World War II, 14–15, 61–62, 78, 98,
  107, 141, 161–62, 163

Yaffe, Martin, 197
Yamanaka factors, 216–17
Yang, Jae-Hyun, 217
yogurt, 113–14

Zhao, Min, 180

www.ingramcontent.com/pod-product-compliance
Lightning Source LLC
Chambersburg PA
CBHW022045020426
42335CB00012B/554